DASH DIET:

THE COMPLETE GUIDE

2 Books in **1**:
DASH Diet for Beginners, Your 21-Day Meal Plan
&
Cookbook With 140 of the Greatest DASH Diet Recipes
to Make You Lose Weight and Lower Your Blood
Pressure

BEATRICE MORELLI

TABLE OF CONTENTS
DASH DIET FOR BEGINNERS

INTRODUCTION 9

CHAPTER 1 WHAT THE DASH DIET IS **11**

CHAPTER 2 HEALTH BENEFITS............................**19**

CHAPTER 3 DASH DIET AND HEALTH **21**

CHAPTER 4 THE IMPORTANCE OF EXERCISE DURING DIET **26**

CHAPTER 5 HOW CAN YOU GET STARTED? **31**

CHAPTER 6 WHAT SHOULD YOU EAT? WHAT SHOULDN'T YOU EAT? THE DO'S AND THE DON'TS **38**

CHAPTER 7 ADVANTAGES AND DISADVANTAGES OF THE DASH DIET **47**

CHAPTER 8 MYTHS ABOUT THE DASH DIET **53**

CHAPTER 9 21 DAY MEAL PLAN.......................... **59**

CHAPTER 10 IMPLEMENTING THE DASH DIET IN YOUR LIFE.. **61**

CHAPTER 11 LOSING WEIGHT WITH DASH DIET... **66**

CONCLUSION...................................... **73**

INTRODUCTION................................ **76**

TABLE OF CONTENTS
DASH DIET COOKBOOK FOR BEGINNERS

CHAPTER 1 HEALTH BENEFITS AND WHY IT WORKS **77**

CHAPTER 2 DASH DIET TIPS......................**81**

CHAPTER 3 BEST DIET TIPS TO LOSE WEIGHT AND IMPROVE HEALTH **84**

CHAPTER 4 BREAKFAST RECIPES **92**

Sweet Potatoes with Coconut Flakes 92
Flaxseed & Banana Smoothie.............................92
Fruity Tofu Smoothie 92
French Toast with Applesauce 93
Banana-Peanut Butter 'n Greens Smoothie 93
Baking Powder Biscuits 94
Oatmeal Banana Pancakes with Walnuts 94
Creamy Oats, Greens & Blueberry Smoothie 95
Banana & Cinnamon Oatmeal 95
Bagels Made Healthy 96
Cereal with Cranberry-Orange Twist 96
No Cook Overnight Oats....................................97
Avocado Cup with Egg 97
Mediterranean Toast 98
Instant Banana Oatmeal 98
Almond Butter-Banana Smoothie 98
Brown Sugar Cinnamon Oatmeal......................99
Buckwheat Pancakes with Vanilla Almond Milk .99
Tomato Bruschetta with Basil..........................100
Sweet Corn Muffins...100
Scrambled Eggs with Mushrooms and Spinach .101
Chia and Oat Breakfast Bran...........................101
Faux Breakfast Hash Brown Cups 102
Maple Mocha Frappe..102
Breakfast Oatmeal in Slow Cooker 103
Apple Cinnamon Overnight Oats 103
Spinach Mushroom Omelette 104
Muesli Scones 104
Sweet Potato Waffles..105
Ezekiel Bread French Toast 106
Mushroom Spinach Omelet 106

CHAPTER 5 LUNCH RECIPES...........................**108**

Veggie Quesadillas 108
Chicken Wraps 108

Black Bean Patties with Cilantro.....................109
Lunch Rice Bowls 110
Salmon Salad 110
Stuffed Mushrooms Caps.................................111
Tuna Salad 111
Shrimp Lunch Rolls 111
Turkey Sandwich with Mozzarella 112
Veggie Soup...112
Avocado and Melon Salad 113
Spaghetti Squash And Sauce 113
Sausage with Potatoes......................................114
Beef Soup 114
Shrimp Salad 115
Watercress, Asparagus And Shrimp Salad 115
Chicken Tacos..116
Millet Cakes 116
Lentils Dal with Yogurt 117
Lunch Quinoa And Spinach Salad 117
Italian Pasta with Parmesan 118
Glazed Ribs..119
Chinese Chicken 119
Chicken and Barley 120
Instant Pot Potato Salad 120
Instant Pot Beef Gyros.....................................121
Instant Pot Lasagna Hamburger Helper 122
Pasta with Meat sauce 122
Tavern Sandwiches in Instant Pot 122
Instant Pot Egg Sandwiches 123
Instant Pot Shredded Chicken 123
Teriyaki Chicken..124
Buffalo Chicken Quinoa bowls........................125
Chicken Tacos..125
Tuscan Chicken Pasta 126
Pork Carnitas...126
Instant Pot Chipotle Burritos 127

CHAPTER 6 DINNER RECIPES.................... **129**

Spinach Rolls 129
Goat Cheese Fold-Overs 129
Crepe Pie 130
Coconut Soup 131
Fish Tacos 131
Cobb Salad 132

CHEESE SOUP 132
TUNA TARTARE 133
CLAM CHOWDER.. 133
ASIAN BEEF SALAD 133
CARBONARA.. 134
CAULIFLOWER SOUP WITH SEEDS 135
PROSCIUTTO-WRAPPED ASPARAGUS 135
STUFFED BELL PEPPERS 136
STUFFED EGGPLANTS WITH GOAT CHEESE.............. 136
KORMA CURRY 137
ZUCCHINI BARS.. 138
MUSHROOM SOUP.. 138
STUFFED PORTOBELLO MUSHROOMS..................... 139
LETTUCE SALAD 139
LEMON GARLIC SALMON 140
CHICKPEA CURRY 140
INSTANT POT CHICKEN THIGHS WITH OLIVES AND CAPERS
.... 141
INSTANT POT SALMON 142
INSTANT POT MAC N' CHEESE............................ 142
INSTANT POT MEDITERRANEAN CHICKEN 143
GREEN CHICKEN AND RICE BOWL 143
TURKEY MEATBALLS WITH SPAGHETTI SQUASH 144
INSTANT POT CHICKEN PARMESAN 145
INSTANT POT CHICKEN MARSALA......................... 145
INSTANT POT SAUSAGE CHICKEN CASSEROLE 146
SPICY PASTA.. 147

CHAPTER 7 DESSERT RECIPES............................148

HEARTY CASHEW AND ALMOND BUTTER.................. 148
THE REFRESHING NUTTER 148
ELEGANT CRANBERRY MUFFINS 149
APPLE AND ALMOND MUFFINS 149
STYLISH CHOCOLATE PARFAIT 150
SUPREME MATCHA BOMB 150
MESMERIZING AVOCADO AND CHOCOLATE PUDDING 150
HEARTY PINEAPPLE PUDDING 151
HEALTHY BERRY COBBLER................................... 151
TASTY POACHED APPLES..................................... 152

HOME MADE TRAIL MIX FOR THE TRIP 152
HEART WARMING CINNAMON RICE PUDDING 153
PURE AVOCADO PUDDING 153
SWEET ALMOND AND COCONUT FAT BOMBS 153
SPICY POPPER MUG CAKE.................................. 154
THE MOST ELEGANT PARSLEY SOUFFLÉ EVER 154
FENNEL AND ALMOND BITES 155
FEISTY COCONUT FUDGE 155
NO BAKE CHEESECAKE 156
EASY CHIA SEED PUMPKIN PUDDING 156
LOVELY BLUEBERRY PUDDING.............................. 157
DECISIVE LIME AND STRAWBERRY POPSICLE 157
RAVAGING BLUEBERRY MUFFIN 158
THE COCONUT LOAF 158
FRESH FIGS WITH WALNUTS AND RICOTTA.............. 159
AUTHENTIC MEDJOOL DATE TRUFFLES 159
TASTY MEDITERRANEAN PEANUT ALMOND BUTTER
POPCORNS.. 160
JUST A MINUTE WORTH MUFFIN........................... 160
HEARTY ALMOND BREAD.................................... 161
LEMON GRANITA 161
LOW CARB BLACKBERRY ICE CREAM 162
CHOCOLATE COCONUT ICE CREAM 162
CHOCOLATE PEPPERMINT POPSICLES 163
PERFECT STRAWBERRY ICE CREAM......................... 163
RASKOLNIKOV VANILLA ICE CREAM....................... 164
TRADITIONAL SPANISH COLD CREAM WITH WALNUTS 164
CHOCOLATE ICE CREAM...................................... 165
AVOCADO AND STRAWBERRIES SALAD.................... 165
BLUEBERRY CREAM 166
APPLE CUPCAKES 166
CINNAMON APPLES 166
VANILLA PUMPKIN BARS 167
COLD CASHEW AND BERRY CAKE 167
CARROT AND MANDARINS COLD CAKE 168

CONCLUSION...169

DASH DIET FOR BEGINNERS:

LEARN HOW THE 21-DAY DASH DIET MEAL PLAN IS PROVEN TO MAKE YOU LOSE WEIGHT AND LOWER YOUR BLOOD PRESSURE. IMPROVE YOUR HEALTH AND LIVE A BETTER LIFE.

BEATRICE MORELLI

Introduction

Thank you for choosing this guide, you will learn everything you need to know about dash diet as a beginner; after this, kindly proceed to my recipe cookbook for delicious and easy to make recipes, *"DASH Diet Cookbook for Beginners: 140 of the Greatest DASH Diet Recipes Designed to Make You Lose Weight and Lower Your Blood Pressure. Unconventional Dishes to Start Enjoying Healthy Food."*

I'm sure you've been through diets in your life. If not you, you must have known people who begin a diet enthusiastically, then hit a plateau and give it all up in frustration and resume their unhealthy eating habits. Wondering what the DASH diet is all about? It's a one of a kind diet, specifically designed to reduce blood pressure levels in people. Hypertension, or high blood pressure, is one of the greatest silent killers of this century.

DASH stands for Dietary Approaches to Stop Hypertension. The DASH diet is rich in fruits, vegetables, whole grains, and low-fat dairy products. Its emphasis isn't on deprivation, but on adaptation. The DASH diet aims to change the way people look at food, to educate them about their bodies, and to teach them to make healthy, sustainable choices.

The DASH diet was created to change lives by changing lifestyles. Unlike more restrictive diets, the DASH diet was designed to be approachable, and to be readily incorporated into people's lives. For the most part, you do not need to shop at special grocery stores or go through agonizing transition periods; you just need to start adjusting your food patterns, one step at a time.

The basics of the DASH diet are simple: Eat more fruits, vegetables, whole grains, and lean protein, and eat less saturated fat, salt, and sweets. It's a common-sense approach to health that really works.

The DASH diet works because it's a lifestyle that can be sustained easily, not a traditional diet. The word "diet" conjures thoughts of temporary deprivation, but the DASH diet is the opposite. It aims at educating individuals on how they can undertake clean or proper eating, on a daily basis, so that they build healthy bodies. Rather than impose strict controls on food content, such as the total number of fat, DASH diet follows important rules of choosing clean foods. When individuals understand the implications of their daily dietary decision making, they're much more likely to choose wisely. Therefore, it is easy to adopt the DASH diet.

The ultimate goal of the DASH diet is to reduce the intake of harmful foods and to choose healthy substitutes instead. When you understand the damage that bad food does to your body, it makes you far less interested in eating it. And once you wean yourself from excess fat, cholesterol, sodium, and sugar, you will be amazed by how much better you feel! Bad food takes its toll in so many ways, not just silently with hypertension and heart disease, but also outwardly in your appearance, energy level, and enthusiasm for life. If you are feeling sluggish, consider what you last ate. Was it good for you? Or bad? Unless you are fueling your body with good food, it will fail you. The DASH diet isn't a strict dietary regimen, but rather a new way of seeing, appreciating, and consuming food.

Grains, vegetables, fruits, low-fat dairy products, seeds, nuts, and lean meat all form the base of the DASH diet. So, there are no strict restrictions, only amazing benefits. Besides giving you a way of turning to healthy eating habits, the DASH diet is primarily known for showing great results in lowering high blood pressure. This diet is rich in several minerals like calcium, zinc, iron, manganese, and potassium, and these nutrients primarily help to regulate the blood pressure. Also, the diet is low in saturated fat and cholesterol but provides a significant amount of protein, which can also help people suffering from high blood pressure.

Knowing what kind of foods make the foundation of this diet makes it clear that it can also be used to lose weight and excess fat. Following this kind of diet means losing about 500 calories a day. Combine that with exercise, and you will get slim fast. What supports this is also the fact that the DASH diet, rich in protein and fiber, keeps you satiated for longer periods and thus prevents overeating and gaining weight.

The DASH diet is one of the few diets that can help you meet your daily requirement for potassium, which, besides countering the effect of salt to raise blood pressure, also helps in preventing osteoporosis. This diet also provides sufficient amounts of vitamin B 12, calcium, and fiber, which are required for proper cell metabolism, building and maintaining strong bones, keeping blood sugar levels stable, and preventing obesity.

Chapter 1 What the DASH diet is

DASH stands for Dietary Approaches to Stop Hypertension. This diet was specifically designed with a mind toward people who suffer from hypertension (high blood pressure). When you dive into the statistics, it is actually quite shocking how destructive this condition is. The American Heart and Stroke Association stated in 2013 that 1 in every 3 American adults suffers with high blood pressure. This is a staggering statistic and indicates that something has to be done about it. This was a chief motivator behind the conceptualization of the DASH diet.

High blood pressure affects the heart negatively and may lead to heart attacks and strokes. Since hypertension does not discriminate and all people can suffer from it, the good news is that every person can do something about it.

The diet is high in fruits, vegetables and lean proteins and restricts red meat, salt, added sugars and fat. This is the diet's main premise and why it is so healthy for you. The table below gives a brief overview of how you should be eating on the DASH diet.

Food Group	Number of servings per day
Whole grains	6-8
Lean meats, poultry and fish	Less than 6
Vegetables	4-5
Fruit	4-5
Dairy (low -fat)	2-3
Fats and oils	2-3
Sodium (salt)	2300mg (1 tsp)
	Number of servings per week
Nuts, seeds and legumes	4-5
Added sugar and candy	Less than 5

Source: West, H. (2018, October 17)

Benefits Of Using The DASH Diet

A diet held in such high esteem must have many benefits. When it comes to health and taking care of yourself, every person looks for what will be the most helpful and yield the most benefits. Luckily the DASH diet holds multiple benefits in various areas.

Lowers blood pressure

Lowering blood pressure is the main reason this diet was conceived. The reason hypertension is so common in western society is the amount of processed and preserved foods we consume. If any average person were to open their kitchen cupboard or their fridge, they would see a large amount of canned goods, processed meats, frozen meals and various other types of foods that have come far from their original state.

In order to preserve food, salt is commonly added to it since salt is a preservative. So anything that is not fresh is most likely to have an unhealthy amount of salt in it. The DASH diet addresses this factor by emphasizing the consumption of whole foods rather than processed foods. If you cook the food yourself, then you will be able to control the amount of salt in it. You can see what you are adding, and there is no risk of any additional unhealthy ingredients.

High blood pressure is bad for our hearts, and we all know our hearts are a vital organ in our bodies. It should be our priority to keep our hearts healthy. The pressure exerted on the heart by hypertension puts an amount of strain on the heart that it is simply not built to handle.

Weight loss

Although not directly what the diet was designed for, this method of eating has been shown to directly impact weight loss. Losing weight will also directly impact your blood pressure since being overweight increases your blood pressure. If you do suffer from hypertension and have been to see a doctor, chances are that you have been advised to lose weight. The DASH diet kills two birds with one stone since you can lower your blood pressure and lose weight all on the same eating plan.

With any diet, in order to lose weight, you have to eat less calories than you are using. The DASH diet already cuts out many high-calorie foods that are high in saturated and total fats as well as added sugars. You will replace these empty calories with comprehensively nutritious foods. This means that the volume of food you eat will be able to sustain you without any increase in your calorie intake since you will be consuming more effective fuel.

Increased nutritional value

Since you will be cutting out empty calories and replacing them with food of a high nutritional value, the amount of vitamins and minerals you will be absorbing into your body will be much higher. Your body will be able to use these nutrients to fight common illnesses, such as the flu and help your body run at an optimal level. You will experience a higher level of energy and endurance throughout the day and when you are exercising. Can you imagine how much healthier a lifestyle that will produce overall?

TYPES OF DASH DIETS

Generally, there are two types of the DASH diet that you'll come across.

- Standard DASH Diet

- Lower Sodium DASH Diet

Standard DASH Diet: With this DASH diet, the sodium intake should exceed 2300 mg per day. This diet is ideal for people who have normal blood pressure.

Lower Sodium DASH Diet: With this DASH diet, the sodium intake must be limited to less than 1500 mg on a daily basis. This DASH diet is suitable for people who are suffering from hypertension (high blood pressure).

Both of these DASH diets have the same goal, to limit salt consumption, because this helps to regulate blood pressure. Moreover, both of the diets also aid in losing weight.

Choosing either one of the two diets depends on your weight and body needs. Your doctor or nutritionist might recommend anywhere from 1,200 to 3,000 or more calories in a day. Therefore, it is vital to identify the right amount of calories that can satisfy your body's needs. Hence, it is wise to consult a nutritionist before starting this diet.

THE DASH DIETARY PROGRAM

Normally, the DASH diet includes the following nutrients, and they should be consumed in the following amounts on a daily basis:

- Saturated fat: 6% of calories

- Protein:18% of calories

- Carbohydrate: 55% of calories

- Total fat: 27% of calories

- Cholesterol: 150 mg

- Sodium: 2,300 mg

- Potassium: 4,700 mg

- Calcium: 1,250 mg

- Magnesium: 500 mg

- Fiber: 30g

In short, a DASH diet is:

- Low in saturated and trans fats

- Rich in fiber, protein, magnesium, calcium and potassium

- Low in sodium

Fats

A lot of people consider fats as the prime culprit for a number of chronic diseases. It's true, but further research has shown that fats are categorized into two types: good fats and bad fats.

Good fats benefit us in many ways. They help reduce inflammation, offer vital fatty acids, and improve our health.

Consuming foods that have good fats is linked to increasing HDL and reducing small dense LDL particles. You can find many foods that are loaded with good fats in the DASH diet, such as:

- Avocados

- Nuts

- Hemp Seeds

- Flax seeds

- Olive oil

- Fish (Rich in omega-3 fatty acids)

Speaking of bad fats, these include vegetable shortening, margarine, hydrogenated vegetable oils (partially) etc. Such foods are said to increase small LDL particles, which can lead to atherogenesis (artery wall disorder).

Fats are vital in any diet, which is why they need to be consumed in moderation. However, on the DASH diet, it is important to carefully choose serving sizes, that is, choose foods that have more good fats and less of the bad fats.

Saturated fat is bad fat and can be found in fatty meat, coconut oil, palm oil, full-fat dairy products and palm kernel oil. Hence, they should be consumed less.

Unsaturated fat is good fat that helps to reduce levels of cholesterol and minimize the risk of heart attacks. Unsaturated fats can be found in olives, avocados, nuts, certain fish, etc.

Proteins

The DASH diet recommends that protein should be consumed in abundance, as it has many health benefits. Protein can be obtained by eating legumes, soy products, nuts, seeds, fish, lean meat, eggs, low-fat dairy, etc.

Processed meats should be avoided because they are linked to hypertension. Some processed meats have also been found to contain carcinogens, which are deadly for our health.

Carbohydrates

In addition to protein, the DASH diet also emphasizes carbs. This is because carbs provide us with energy and many micronutrients that help regulate many body functions.

There are many diets that suggest dieters should reduce carb intake, as this increases calorie consumption. However, this is an unhealthy approach and can lead to poor health and digestive issues as well.

The food in the DASH diet is rich in carbs, and includes:

- Low glycemic index fruits.

- Green vegetables – spinach, kale, broccoli, collards, mustards.

- Whole grains – cracked wheat, millets, oats.

- Beans and legumes.

Other Nutrients

There are many other nutrients that are essential for the body and must be consumed. The DASH diet recommends calcium, magnesium and potassium. Foods that are rich in these nutrients help fight endothelial dysfunction and enhance smooth muscle relaxation.

- Potassium: bananas, oranges and spinach.

- Calcium: dairy products and green vegetables.

- Magnesium: whole grains, leafy vegetables, nuts and seeds.

MICRONUTRIENTS IN THE DASH DIET

The DASH diet is all about the right portion sizes, eating nutrient-rich foods and making sure that the amounts are as per the guidelines.

There's no doubt that the DASH diet's main goal is to help reduce blood pressure, but it also helps with weight loss. It does so by reducing the cholesterol level and making sure that diabetes is controlled.

According to The National Kidney Foundation, people with kidney diseases should go on the DASH diet. This is because it incorporates less sodium and increases the intake of healthy nutrients such as magnesium, calcium and potassium. This helps lower blood pressure.

According to The United States Department of Agriculture (USDA) the DASH diet is the ideal eating plan for all Americans.

Some people consider the DASH diet to be a vegetarian diet, but it's not. It does incorporate many fruits and vegetables, non-fat dairy foods, beans, nuts and other nutritious items because of the healthy benefits they provide us with. But, it also includes meat and fish.

The DASH diet also recommends that dieters steer clear of junk and processed food, as these are loaded with too much sodium, which not only spikes blood pressure but also contributes to weight gain.

Let's get to know about the micronutrients that can be found in the DASH diet and how they help:

•   Potassium: Fruit are loaded with potassium, and potassium is linked to reducing blood pressure.

•   Unsaturated Fats: These are good fats and help to reduce bad cholesterol levels.

•   Omega-3 Fatty Acids: Too much fat in the blood can disrupt the heart's rhythm, and lead to heart attacks. According to studies, omega-3 helps to reduce triglyceride levels (fats in the blood). This way the risk of heart attack is reduced.

•   Fiber: Helps to suppress our appetite and control calorie intake.

•   L-arginine: Helps improve the functionality of the artery walls by promoting flexibility and reducing the risk of blood clots.

•   Carbs: Energy provider.

Role of Fruit in the DASH Diet

•   The DASH diet recommends eating a lot of fruit, which contain a huge amount of useful nutrients that aid in reducing blood pressure and weight.

For example, potassium is one of our most important nutrients as it helps to balance the electrolytes in our bodies. Bananas contain a high level of potassium. There is 358 mg potassium in 100 grams of a banana.

According to this study, consuming two bananas on a daily basis for two weeks can help reduce blood pressure by 10%.

•   Then there are citrus fruits, which include grapefruit, oranges, lemons and limes. These are ideal fruit on the DASH diet, thanks to the low amount of sodium they contain. In fact, there are many essential vitamins and minerals in this fruit. For example, oranges alone contain 326 mg of potassium, and avocados contain 690 mg of potassium.

•   Apart from potassium, there are many other nutrients that also benefit our bodies in various ways. A Florida State University study says that watermelon aids in regulating blood pressure, as it contains a high amount of L-citrulline (an amino acid that processes L-arginine and improves blood circulation). The same study also says that L-citrulline also helps in reducing high blood pressure.

•   Another study published in The American Journal of Clinical Nutrition says that fruit such as blueberries, strawberries, cranberries, blackcurrants and oranges contain anthocyanins. This provides protection against high blood pressure.

So, the DASH diet emphasizes that lots of fruit should be included in the diet because they help control blood pressure, weight loss, and provide other health benefits as well.

THE IMPORTANCE OF INCLUDING MINERALS

The reason that the DASH diet is a complete diet is because it is balanced. It won't ask you to cut out carbs, fats or any nutrient completely. It's a diet plan that is offered to individuals, based on their bodies.

The DASH diet focuses a great deal on nutrient intake because they help in many ways.

Importance of Potassium: Potassium counteracts the effects of sodium and helps control blood pressure.

One major benefit of including fruit and vegetables in your diet is that they help control blood pressure. Fruit such as oranges, citrus fruit, bananas, apples, avocados, raisins and apricots are high in potassium.

Note: Canned or processed fruit aren't as healthy as fresh fruit because most of the potassium is washed away during the process. Fruit should be eaten fresh or frozen.

Apart from fruit, leafy green vegetables such as parsley, lettuce, broccoli, peas, spinach, potatoes, lima beans and tomatoes are also full of potassium.

Whole grains also make the list of high potassium yielding fruit. These include wheat germ, seeds and nuts.

Fish is another source of potassium that you can enjoy on the DASH diet. Sardines, cod, flounder and salmon are rich in potassium. Calcium: Needed to build and maintain strong bones. The National Heart, Lung, and Blood Institute (NHLBI) recommends including foods that are rich in calcium. People who opt for a 1,600 calorie diet should consume at least two 8-ounce servings of low-fat milk/yogurt or fat-free milk. If you're following a 2,600 calorie diet then three servings of 8 ounces each needs to be taken.

The daily recommendation of calcium for a healthy adult is 1,000 milligrams. However, the NHLBI suggests increasing the amount of calcium to around 1250 mg.

Foods that are rich in calcium include dairy products (yogurt and milk). Cheese is also allowed but not in abundance because it also contains sodium.

Milk and yogurt are healthy for the body, as they are easily absorbed.

One glass (8 ounces) of milk will give you about 300 mg of calcium and 8 ounces of yogurt will provide between 250 mg to 350 mg of calcium. You can also take calcium-fortified orange juice, as it will provide you with 300 mg of calcium. Calcium-fortified orange juice will also provide you with potassium. Magnesium: It is recommended that healthy individuals have at least 400 mg of magnesium each day, because it helps a number of functions and helps process many chemical reactions in the body as well. Magnesium helps reduce blood pressure, triggers an anti-inflammatory response in the body and also has many other benefits. Dark Chocolate: Dark chocolate has many benefits. It improves blood flow, adds shine to the skin, and makes you look good. Plus, it contains magnesium, which is good for your health. A 28 gram piece of dark chocolate (1 ounce) can provide you with 64 mg of magnesium.

Besides magnesium, dark chocolate contains other nutrients as well, including iron, manganese and copper. Other than that, it contains some prebiotic fibers that also help feed the healthy bacteria in your gut.

That's not all; it also contains antioxidants that help neutralize harmful free radicals that can cause dangerous diseases.

Dark chocolate also helps to maintain a healthy heart because it is loaded with flavonoids, which is an antioxidant compound that helps prevent "bad" LDL cholesterol from oxidizing and narrowing your arteries.

Dark chocolate that has 70% cocoa is what you should choose, as it has added benefits.

Avocado: Another amazing source of magnesium is avocado. One avocado a day provides 15% of daily magnesium requirements (58 mg).

This fruit contains several nutrients, including potassium, B vitamins and vitamin K. Moreover, it is also an excellent source of fiber. Fiber is quite beneficial for a number of things such as regulating blood pressure, improving bowel movements, etc.

Moreover, eating an avocado can suppress your appetite, improve blood sugar levels, and also lower inflammation in the body.

Nuts: Almonds, cashews, Brazil nuts, etc., are loaded with magnesium. Eating one ounce of cashews alone can provide 20% of the recommended daily intake of nuts, as it contains 82 mg of magnesium. Other than that, it also contains fiber and monounsaturated fats. Both of these help to control blood pressure and reduce cholesterol levels in people who are suffering from diabetes.

Moreover, Brazil nuts are said to contain higher amounts of selenium, which are linked with many health benefits, such as reducing the risk of heart disease and cancer.

Eating two Brazil nuts daily can keep you in good shape.

Brazil nuts make a great snack food and will provide you with amazing nutrients that will help your body.

Chapter 2 Health benefits

The DASH diet is particularly suggested for individuals with hypertension (high blood pressure) or prehypertension. The DASH diet-eating plan has been demonstrated to lower blood pressure in considers supported by the National Institutes of Health (Dietary Approaches to Stop Hypertension). Notwithstanding being a low salt (or low sodium) plan, the DASH diet gives extra benefits to lessen blood pressure. It depends on an eating plan wealthy in fruits and vegetables, and low fat or non-fat dairy, with whole grains. It is a high fiber, low to direct fat diet, rich in potassium, calcium, and magnesium.

Who can benefit?

Individuals who follow the DASH diet can lessen levels of:

• Blood pressure

• Blood sugar

• Triglycerides, or fat, in the blood

• Low-thickness lipoprotein (LDL), or "terrible" cholesterol

• Insulin obstruction

These are, for the most part, highlights of metabolic disorder, a condition that likewise includes weight, type 2 diabetes, and a greater danger of cardiovascular illness.

Some Proven Benefits of the DASH Diet

A few preliminaries have been completed to help recognize and evaluate the benefits of the DASH diet. These include:

• Reduction in blood pressure - in only two weeks of following the DASH diet, the blood pressure frequently drops a couple of focuses, and whenever persevered in, this could bring about the systolic blood pressure descending by eight to fourteen focuses.

• The DASH diet additionally improves bone quality and forestalls osteoporosis due to expanded calcium consumption from dairy items and verdant green vegetables.

• A high admission of new or solidified fruits and vegetables is related to a lower danger of disease in the long haul.

• The metabolic issues, for example, cardiovascular ailment and diabetes, just as cerebrovascular illness, are diminished by the reasonable food admission with the DASH diet, prompting lowered fat utilization and expanded substitution of complex starches for straightforward sugars. This prompts an abatement in the aggregate and LDL cholesterol in the blood, just as a reduction in blood pressure.

• A lowered danger of gout by lessening corrosive uric levels in subjects with hyperuricemia is an extra advantage of the DASH diet.

Subsequently, the DASH diet is not an accident or hardship diet yet one that allows for complete nutrition and long haul foundation of healthy eating. To diminish sodium utilization, even more, a low sodium variant of the DASH diet is likewise accessible. This decreases sodium to 1500 mg daily from the standard 2300 mg/day, which itself is a significant enhancement for the normal American diet.

Applicable Trials Showing Benefit of the DASH Diet

The DASH preliminary found that this diet realized lower blood pressure and LDL cholesterol contrasted and the normal American diet, either in that capacity or with added fruits and vegetables. This preliminary included 459 grown-ups and the DASH diet was contrasted and two others that had a day-by-day sodium admission of 3000 mg.

Different diets spoke to the normal American diet without and with added fruits and vegetables. In any case, none of the dieters followed a veggie-lover plan or one, which included foods that would not be eaten eventually by normal Americans. The DASH diet had the most impact on decreasing blood pressure, while the diet with added products of the soil indicated the middle of the road results. This was found in people who had ordinary or raised blood pressures.

The DASH-Sodium preliminary then again had 412 subjects who followed either the DASH or a run of the American mill diet. Day by day, sodium levels were set at high (3,300 mg), low moderate (2,300 mg), and low (1,500 mg) individually, in every one of these diets. Sodium limitation was constantly found to diminish the blood pressure, yet the impact was more noteworthy with the DASH diet. It could likewise be said that the DASH diet was significantly increasingly successful with sodium limitation.

The PREMIER preliminary had 810 members in three gatherings, the man who got just exhortation; however, no directing for conduct changes; the second was on a setup treatment plan with guiding for a half-year; and the third with a plan, advising and the DASH diet.

While the blood pressure was diminished in each of the three gatherings, the exhortation just gathering had the least weight reduction while the third gathering indicated the most decrease in blood pressure and weight.

Chapter 3 DASH Diet and Health

The DASH Diet was really intended to help people who suffer from high blood pressure levels. By modifying your dietary patterns and choices to consuming delicious yet healthy food, you can keep your blood pressure levels in check. Aside from reducing your sodium intake, the DASH Diet also increases your absorption of Potassium, Magnesium, and Calcium. By following this diet, you will be able to experience a drop on your blood pressure levels to a few points. And if you continually follow this diet regimen, your systolic blood pressure can go down by at the most 8 to 14 points.

DASH Diet and Weight Loss

Because the Dash Diet encourages you to consume only healthy foods, you will be able to reduce your weight over a long time. Since this particular diet encourages you to consume complex carbohydrates and healthy starches, your body will be able to process the starch into glucose and use it up efficiently as an energy source for the body. Moreover, since complex carbohydrates also contain plant materials such as fiber and cellulose that are not digested, they only bulk up on your stomach, thus making you feel full for a longer time. This prevents you from craving for too much food during the day. And since you are consuming foods that are calorie dense but slowly assimilated by the body, you give your body enough time to metabolize the food and utilize it as an energy source.

DASH Diet and Diabetes

Since this particular diet encourages the consumption of healthful carbohydrates in the form of complex carbs, they do not get converted easily into glucose. The types of carbohydrates that are recommended for this diet is very healthy for the body, unlike simple sugars such as table sugar, white rice, and white flour that gets easily converted to glucose. If not utilized by the body, they are converted into fats and stored in the liver. The more fats stored in the body, the more the body becomes tolerant to insulin. This can lead to metabolic diseases such as obesity, non-alcoholic fatty liver disease, and diabetes. The DASH Diet corrects this by making sure that you only consume good carbohydrates.

DASH Diet Leads to A Healthier Kidney

The DASH Diet is supported by the National Kidney Foundation. Hypertension is related to kidney diseases. Since the DASH Diet helps decrease the blood pressure level, it can also help reduce the onset of kidney diseases. The reduced intake of salt and other Sodium-rich foods can help reduce the formation of kidney stones.

DASH Diet and Cholesterol/Heart/Disease/Osteoporosis/Stroke

The DASH Diet comes with a lot of benefits for the body. It is also known to lower down cholesterol level, improve heart health, prevent stroke, and osteoporosis. Because it promotes the consumption of good fats and fatty acid, it can help increase the number of low-density lipoproteins (LDL) in the blood. Good fats also help prevent inflammation. It protects major organs, particularly the cardiovascular system, thereby improving heart health. Having better heart health also prevents the likelihood of stroke. And since the DASH Diet promotes the consumption of micronutrients, including Calcium, it can also help improve bone strength and avoid the early onset of osteoporosis.

Hypertension: How Does Diet Come into Play and Why DASH Diet Works?

Food plays a vital role in the development of hypertension. Studies showed that consumption of foods rich in Sodium (salt), particularly processed food, can increase the likelihood of developing hypertension. But can diet alone help stabilize blood pressure levels? Researchers from the NIH noted that dietary interventions play vital roles in improving the condition of people suffering from different situations. Dietary change can decrease the systolic blood pressure level by about 6 to 11 mmHg. This means that by following the right diet regimen and omitting foods that are not helpful to the blood pressure level can bring relief to hypertensive people.

The DASH Diet was developed by expert nutritionists and has undergone several trials to prove that it can really benefit by reducing the systolic pressure. In fact, the reduction of the systolic blood pressure was observed not only among hypertensive individuals but also those who have normal blood pressure levels.

Tips for Planning Your DASH Diet

The DASH Diet is one of the easiest ways to maintain your healthy lifestyle, thus it does not take rocket science for you to be able to follow and achieve your health goals with this diet. When planning to do the DASH Diet, there are some things that you need to consider first. Below are important tips for planning your DASH Diet.

• Make small changes: Remember that this particular diet regimen encourages you to make diet changes by eating whole foods. Making small changes allow you to adjust to this regimen easily. You can do this by gradually making changes in your diet. For instance, you can add more serving of vegetables every meal or substitute unhealthy dressings with healthier condiments.

• Limit your intake of meat: Start limiting the amount of meat that you are going to take in. If you are currently eating large amounts of meat, you can start cutting back at least two servings every day.

• Start avoiding full-fat options: Start avoiding full-fat options once you start planning to do the DASH Diet. It is easier to omit foods that are not allowed for this particular diet, especially when you started restricting yourself earlier in the first place.

• Practice smart shopping: Shopping is one of the biggest aspects of the DASH Diet. Since your shopping will be restricted to buying whole fresh food, you need to learn how to read food labels and choose items that do not contain any unnecessary additives, particularly salt. This is also the time when you start removing processed foods from your shopping list.

• Start cooking healthy: When you cook your food, try learning how to cook without too much or no salt at all. This may be challenging for you, but you can try experimenting with different salt-free flavorings, herbs, and spices.

• Eat out less often: If you love to eat out all the time, try to minimize your dinner trips once you have started with the DASH Diet. This is especially true if you are still getting the hang of this diet. The problem with eating out is that most restaurants either use too much salt when flavoring their food. If you cannot help but eat out, ask the restaurant to prepare food without added salt or MSG.

• Plan your meals ahead: Another tip to make you successful in your DASH Diet is to plan your meals ahead. Planning your meals weekly is a great way to stick to this diet. A weekly meal plan will also serve as your guide on when to eat and what to eat. This will help you avoid over snacking or eating foods that you are not supposed to eat.

The DASH Diet Food Pyramid

The DASH Diet is a very straight-forward diet regimen, but it still helps especially for starters like you to have a guide. This is where the DASH Diet food pyramid comes in. The DASH Diet pyramid is just like your usual food guide, but it indicates what types of food you can eat for this particular diet regimen with specific serving amounts for a 2000-calorie daily diet. The food pyramid is also carefully designed to reduce the total fat in food choices.

The food items that are listed at the bottom of the pyramid are the fruits and vegetables. They should be consumed at 8 to 10 servings daily. This is followed by whole grains. Both the low-fat and meats are at the third tier of the pyramid, that means you need to consume less of it. The fourth level of the pyramid includes beans, nuts, and seeds. While sweets belong to the top of the pyramid and should be taken with fewer servings weekly. If you notice, there are only three types of food groups that are included in the food pyramid. Below is a short summary of the types of food that you are allowed to eat under the DASH Diet.

• Carbohydrates: Carbohydrates is sourced from different types of foods, including fruits, vegetables, grains, nuts, and seeds. They contain starch and cellulose. The DASH Diet encourages the consumption of healthy starches not only to supply energy for the body but to provide the body with protective micronutrients. Healthy sources of carbohydrates that are recommended for the DASH Diet include green leafy vegetables, whole grains, low glycemic index fruits, legumes, beans, nuts, and seeds.

• Fats: Not all fats are created equally. Good fats can help maintain homeostasis in the body by preventing inflammation. Fats that are good for you are sourced from olive oil, avocadoes, nuts, flaxseed, hempseed, and fish's rich in Omega-3 fatty acids.

• Proteins: Similar to fats, not all proteins are created equally. The DASH Diet recommends more servings of plant-based proteins from legumes, nuts, and seeds. For animal protein, you can only consume lean meats, chicken, turkey, eggs, fish, and low-fat dairy.

DASH Diet Food No-Goes

With the DASH Diet, nothing is technically off-limits, but dieters are recommended to eat less of foods that are bad for the health. But if you are new to this diet, it is crucial that you know about which foods you should avoid and which foods to avoid if you want to be successful in following the DASH Diet.

• Red meat: Red meat is not recommended if you want to follow the DASH Diet. However, you can occasionally eat grass-fed beef as it is high in Omega-3 fatty acid due to its diet.

• Bad fats: As mentioned earlier, not all fats are created equally. Avoid bad fats, including margarine, hydrogenated vegetable oil, and vegetable shortening, because they promote atherogenesis.

• Salt or Sodium: The DASH Diet is a low salt diet or none at all as salt can cause hypertension. Instead of using salt, use the spice rack to improve the flavor of your food.

• Alcohol: Consumption of alcohol can elevate your blood pressure levels. Too much alcohol can eventually damage the liver, brain, and heart. If you cannot avoid but drink alcohol, make sure that you drink one glass if you are a woman and two if you are a man.

• Cured meats: All kinds of cured meats are not recommended because they contain high amounts of Sodium that may cause hypertension. Moreover, cured meats also contain potential carcinogens that can cause cancer.

• Full-fat dairy: The purpose of the DASH Diet is to lessen the intake of fat. This includes full-fat dairy, such as milk, cream, and cheese.

• Other foods: Other foods that are included in the no-eat list include high-fat snacks, sugary sweets or snacks, salad dressings, sauces, and gravies.

Low Sodium Philosophy

Sodium is the culprit of hypertension as it is widely known to increase blood pressure levels. Several studies have backed the dangers of consuming too much salt in your diet. When too much salt is taken in, it causes imbalance as well as reduce the ability of the body to regulate the excretion of fluid by the kidneys.

The American Heart Association released a dietary guideline on the amount of Sodium that an average American should take in. The average American takes in five or more teaspoons of salt daily, while the recommended daily allowance is 1,500 mg per day. This is like taking in 20 times as much as the body needs of salt every day.

It is vital to take note that Sodium is not only found in salt but also in many types of food so if you are not careful about the kinds of food you are going to eat, you are probably eating twice as much Sodium without even knowing it. Large amounts of Sodium are hidden in processed and canned foods. Your fast food favorites are also laden with Sodium. The thing is that if you are not careful with the food that you are eating, you may end up suffering from hypertension and other types of diseases.

The low Sodium philosophy encourages people to consume less salt by minding what they eat. Reading labels is very important so that you will know whether you are consuming too much salt on your food or not. Foods rich in Sodium are those labeled with brine, salt, and monosodium glutamate.

While the DASH Diet encourages people to cook meals from scratch using whole food ingredients, buying pre-packaged meals under this diet is highly unlikely. Under this philosophy, you are encouraged to eat more home-cooked meals because you know how much salt you are putting in your food. But more than food, this particular philosophy also encourages people to avoid using medications that contain high amounts of Sodium, including Alka Seltzer and Bromo Seltzer. The thing is that anything that contains high amounts of Sodium – from food, beverage to medication – should be avoided when following the low Sodium philosophy.

Chapter 4 The Importance Of Exercise During Diet

Exercise is good for human health in many ways, regardless of what you choose to do. My goal in this section is not only to gently introduce you to the numerous health benefits that regular physical activity can offer but also to remind you that your 28-day plan will include a diverse, varied exercise routine that I hope provides options that everyone can get something out of.

Although the DASH diet focuses on food choices, there is no denying that regular and varied exercise represents an important component of a healthy lifestyle and one that can confer additional benefits. For those of you who are starting from square one, you should know that any exercise is better than none and that there is absolutely nothing wrong with starting slowly and easing into a more rigorous routine. With that being said, the CDC identifies moderate intensity aerobic activity that totals 120 to 150 minutes weekly, in combination with two additional weekly days of muscular resistance training, as an ideal combination to confer numerous health benefits to adults. Per the CDC, these benefits include the following:

Better weight management: When combined with dietary modification, regular physical activity plays a role in supporting or enhancing weight-management efforts. Regular exercise is a great way to expend calories on top of any dietary changes you will be making on this program.

Reduced risk for cardiovascular disease: A reduction in blood pressure is a well-recognized benefit of regular physical activity, which ultimately contributes to a reduced risk of cardiovascular disease.

Reduced risk of type 2 diabetes: Regular physical activity is known to improve blood glucose control and insulin sensitivity.

Improved mood: Regular physical activity is associated with improvements in mood and reductions in anxiety owing to the manner in which exercise positively influences the biochemistry of the human brain by releasing hormones and affecting neurotransmitters.

Better sleep: Those who exercise more regularly tend to sleep better than those who don't, which may be partially owing to the reductions in stress and anxiety that often occur in those who exercise regularly.

Stronger bones and muscles: Combining cardiovascular and resistance training confers serious benefits to both your bones and your muscles, which keep your body functioning at a high level as you age.

A longer life span: Those who exercise regularly tend to enjoy a lower risk of chronic disease and a longer life span.

As you will see in the 28-day plan, your recommended exercise totals will be met by exercising four out of the seven days a week. The exercise days will be broken up as follows: All four of the active days will include aerobic exercise for 30 minutes. As a beginner, I encourage you to start slowly and build up to the four days. Two of the four active days will also include strength training. The bottom line is that you don't have to exercise for hours each day to enjoy the health benefits of physical activity. Our goal with this plan is to make the health benefits of exercise as accessible and attainable as possible for those who are ready and willing to give it a try. Before we get to the good stuff, though, there is still a lot of wisdom to be shared about getting the most out of your workouts.

GETTING THE MOST OUT OF YOUR WORKOUTS

Just as with healthy eating strategies, there are certainly important things to keep in mind about physical activity that will help support your long-term success. Let's take a look at a few important considerations that will help you get the most out of your workouts:

Rest days: Even though we haven't even started, I'm going to preach the importance of good rest. Don't forget that you are taking part in this journey to improve your health for the long term, not to burn yourself out in 28 days. Although some of you with more experience with exercise may feel confident going above and beyond, my best advice for the majority of those reading is to listen to your body and take days off to minimize risk of injury and burnout.

Stretching: Stretching is a great way to prevent injury and keep you pain-free both during workouts and in daily life. Whether it's a deliberate activity after a workout or through additional means such as yoga, stretching is beneficial in many ways.

Enjoyment: There is no right or wrong style of exercise. You are being provided a diverse plan that emphasizes a variety of different cardiovascular and resistance training exercises. If there are certain activities within these groups that you don't enjoy, it's okay not to do them. Your ability to stick with regular physical activity in the long term will depend on finding a style of exercise that you enjoy.

Your limits: Physical activity is good for you, and it should be fun, too. It's up to you to keep it that way. While it is important to challenge yourself, don't risk injury by taking things too far too fast.

Your progress: Although this is not an absolute requirement, some of you reading may find joy and fulfillment through tracking your exercise progress and striving toward a longer duration, more repetitions, and so on. If you are the type who enjoys a competitive edge, it may be fun to find a buddy to exercise and progress with.

Warm-ups: Last but certainly not least, your exercise routine will benefit greatly from a proper warm-up routine, which includes starting slowly or doing exercises similar to the ones included in your workout, but at a lower intensity.

SET A ROUTINE

The exercise part of the DASH plan was developed with CDC exercise recommendations in mind in order to support your best health. For some, the 28-day plan may seem like a lot; for others it may not seem like that much. If we look at any exercise routine from a very general perspective, there are at least three broad categories to be aware of.

Strength training: This involves utilizing your muscles against some form of counterweight, which may be your own body or dumbbells. These types of activities alter your resting metabolic rate by supporting the development of muscle while also strengthening your bones.

Aerobic exercise: Also known as cardiovascular activity, these are the quintessential exercises such as jogging or running that involve getting your body moving and getting your heart rate up.

Mobility, flexibility, and balance: Stretching after workouts or even devoting your exercise time on one day a week to stretching or yoga is a great way to maintain mobility and prevent injury in the long term.

This routine recommends involving a combination of both cardiovascular and resistance training. You will be provided with a wide array of options to choose from to accommodate a diverse exercise routine. My best recommendation is to settle on the types of exercises that offer a balance between enjoyment and challenge. Remember that the benefits of physical activity are to be enjoyed well beyond just your 28-day plan, and the best way to ensure that is the case is selecting movements you truly enjoy. My final recommendation in this regard is to also include some form of stretching either after your workouts or on a rest day.

Cardio and Body Weight Exercises

Your 28-day plan will be built around the cardiovascular and strength-training exercises that are detailed in this section. In addition to a variety of different cardiovascular exercise options, the strength-training options you will be provided are divided into four distinct categories: core, lower body, upper body, and full body. Per your sample routine, an ideal strength workout will include one exercise from each of these categories:

CARDIO

Brisk walking: This is essentially walking at a pace beyond your normal walking rate for a purpose beyond just getting from point A to point B.

Jogging: This is the intermediary stage between brisk walking and running and can be used as an accompaniment to either exercise, depending on your fitness level.

Running: The quintessential and perhaps most well-recognized cardiovascular exercise.

Jumping jacks: Although 30 minutes straight of jumping jacks may be impractical, they are a good complement to the other activities on this list.

Dancing: Those who have a background in dancing may enjoy using it to their advantage, but anyone can put on their favorite songs and dance like there's nobody watching.

Jump rope: Own a jump rope? Why not use it as part of your cardiovascular workout? It is a fun way to get your cardio in.

Other options (equipment permitting): Activities like rowing, swimming and water aerobics, biking, and using elliptical and stair climbing machines can be great ways to exercise.

In order to meet the CDC guidelines, your goal will be to work up to a total of 30 minutes of cardiovascular activity per workout session. You may use a combination of the exercises listed. I suggest that beginners should start with brisk walking or jogging—whatever activity you are most comfortable with.

CORE

Plank: The plank is a classic core exercise that focuses on stability and strength of the muscles in the abdominal and surrounding areas. Engage your buttocks, press your forearms into the ground, and hold for 60 seconds. Beginners may start with a 15- to 30-second hold and work their way up.

Side plank: Another core classic and a plank variation that focuses more on the oblique muscles on either side of your central abdominals. Keep the buttocks tight, and prevent your torso from sagging to get the most out of this exercise. Wood chopper: A slightly more dynamic movement that works the rotational functionality of your core and mimics chopping a log of wood. You can start with little to no weight until you feel comfortable and progress from there. Start the move with feet shoulder width apart, back straight, and slightly crouched. If you are using weight, hold it with both hands next to the outside of either thigh, twist to the side, and lift the weight across and upward, keeping your arms straight and turning your torso such that you end up with the weight above your opposite shoulder.

LOWER BODY

Goblet squat: Start your stance with feet slightly wider than shoulder width and a dumbbell held tightly with both hands in front of your chest. Sit back into a squat, hinging at both the knee and the hip joint, and lower your legs until they are parallel to the ground. Push up through your heels to the starting position and repeat. Use a chair to squat onto if you don't feel comfortable.

Dumbbell walking lunge: Start upright with a dumbbell in each hand and feet in your usual standing position. Step forward with one leg and sink down until your back knee is just above the ground. Remain upright and ensure the front knee does not bend over the toes. Push through the heel of the front foot and step forward and through with your rear foot. Start with no weights, and add weight as you feel comfortable.

Romanian dead lift: Unlike the squat and lunge, the Romanian dead lift puts the primary emphasis on the rear muscles of the legs (hamstrings). Stand in a similar starting position to walking lunges, but this time you will hinge at the hips and push your buttocks and hip backward while naturally lowering the dumbbells in front of you. Squeeze your buttocks on the ascent back to the starting position. You can also do this exercise on one leg to improve balance and increase core activation—however, you may need to use lighter weights.

UPPER BODY

Push-ups: These are the ultimate body-weight exercise and can be done just about anywhere. You will want to set up with your hands just beyond shoulder width, keeping your body in a straight line and always engaging your core as you ascend and descend, without letting your elbows flare out. Those who struggle to perform push-ups consecutively can start by performing them on their knees or even against a wall if regular push-ups sound like too much. Dumbbell shoulder press: A great exercise for upper-body and shoulder strength. Bring a pair of dumbbells to ear level, palms forward, and straighten your arms overhead.

FULL BODY

Mountain climbers: On your hands and feet, keep your body in a straight line, with your abdominal and buttocks muscles engaged, similar to the top position of a push-up. Rapidly alternate pulling your knees into your chest while keeping your core tight. Continue in this left, right, left, right rhythm as if you are replicating a running motion. Always try to keep your spine in a straight line. Push press: This is essentially a combination move incorporating a partial squat and a dumbbell shoulder press. Using a weight that you are comfortable with, stand feet slightly beyond shoulder width, with light dumbbells held in a pressing position. Descend for a squat to a depth you feel comfortable with, and on the ascent simultaneously push the dumbbells overhead. Burpee (advanced/optional): This is a classic full-body exercise that is essentially a dynamic combination of a push-up, a squat, and a jump. This particular exercise is very effective but may be challenging for some and should be utilized only by those who feel comfortable. The proper sequencing of the movement involves starting from a standing position before lowering into a squat, placing your hands on the floor, and jumping backward to land on the balls of your feet while keeping your core strong. Jump back to your hands and jump again into the air, reaching your hands upward.

Stay Hydrated

Proper hydration by drinking water is an important habit that supports good health and weight management. Caloric drinks with minimal nutrients, like soda, have become an increasingly common source of calories in our population, and replacing such beverages with plain drinking water is a valuable step to take toward better health. Using natural flavors like a splash of lemon is a good way to transition from drinking sweetened beverages to plain water. It is recommended that women drink about 11 cups a day and men drink about 14 cups a day. Keep in mind that this includes fluid from both foods and beverages, not just water. Certain types of food, especially fruit and certain vegetables, have very high water contents. Beverages such as coffee, tea, and carbonated water also count toward your daily totals. Drinking enough water will also help prevent constipation and work together with the fiber from your diet to keep your bowels working effectively.

Chapter 5 How can you get started?

While it may be appealing to ignore the preparation phase and just dive directly into a diet, it's crucial to spend some time on how incorporating DASH into your meal plan will impact every aspect of your life. Smart preparation is among the best methods to make sure you're successful with the DASH Diet plan. Usually, you may think to plan the meals of yours just on special events like holidays, birthdays and social gatherings but changing like this of thinking and producing both short-term and long-term diet plans will reduce the probability that you will fall back into older, harmful eating patterns. You would not venture out on a very long road trip without having a map or maybe GPS system, so the reason joins a trip as important as this without forethought.

When you eat is equally as important as what you consume. Planning mealtimes and also snack times can help make sure your body remains fueled and doesn't enter calorie conservation mode.

Begin the day of yours with a large breakfast like a treat approximately 2 hours before lunch and also have a different treat approximately 2 hours before dinner. It might sound counter intuitive in the beginning but try making dinner probably the smallest food of the day instead of the largest and also make a routine of refusing to eat for a minimum of 3 hours before bedtime. This particular way, your body utilizes the foods eating instead of keeping it as fat.

What is Your Motivation?

To achieve success with the DASH Diet regime, it is crucial to understand why you would like to be better or weigh less. Before getting started, invest time thinking about the reasons of yours for beginning this program along with considering your commitment level:

•Is my inspiration coming from an external source or am I self motivated?

•Am I prepared for this program?

•What in case setbacks occur? Exactly how will I cope with them?

•Am I dedicated to make the required changes?

•Is my family dedicated to support me? In case not, why don't you?

Determine Your BMI and Weight

Before starting up the DASH Diet, it is crucial to understand the weight of yours as well as your entire body mass index (BMI). In case you have not stepped on a scale for many years, this is the time to get it done. You might also need to evaluate calves, upper arms, thighs, chest, hips and your waist before starting the plan because these dimensions will serve as another way for monitoring success.

Decide on a method for capturing the statistics of yours or maybe have a totally free online weight tracker or perhaps smartphone app before taking the first set of measurements.

Start by checking out the weight and intend to weigh yourself each week at about the same time on a set day; for instance, you are able to decide to weigh yourself each Wednesday early morning before breakfast.

Once you obtain your starting weight, do the dinner table on the right to determine the BMI of yours.

Round the weight of yours up or down to probably the nearest ten pounds; then check out the stage in which that quantity intersects with the height of yours. For instance, in case you weigh 200 lbs and you're 5 feet 6 inches tall, your BMI is thirty two.

Then, understand your BMI:

Under 18.5: Underweight

18.5-24: Normal weight

24-29: Overweight

Thirty or even higher: Obese

In case you belong within the obese category, figure out what the level of being overweight is:

30-34: Class I obesity

35-39: Class II obesity

Forty or even higher: Class III obesity

Regardless of the BMI of yours, so however alarmed you might think at the numbers which appear on the scale, it is crucial you view these figures as a place to start instead as purpose for discouragement. You will probably find it beneficial to remind yourself that you're simply one of the about 50 percent of Americans that are heavy.

Anything you do, do not get caught in the hole of berating yourself for everything you see before you. Indeed, some actions or maybe inaction did contribute to those numbers, though it's essential to concentrate on the place you're going instead of to defeat yourself up about the place you have been.

Eliminate Undesirable Foods as well as Sources of Temptation

When you've calculated your BMI and weight, along with other measurements, it is time to remove sources of temptation. The ideal place to start is in your house pantry and refrigerator.

Begin by reading labels. Foods that have a high percent of sodium, high-fructose corn syrup or hydrogenated fat or even partially hydrogenated fats must be removed immediately, including:

•Potato chips, other salty snack and pretzels foods

•Packaged deli meats

•Dry cereals with sugars, artificial coloring along with additional additives

•Canned goods including beans and vegetables unless they're low-sodium

•Frozen pizzas, prepackaged meals, jarred sauces and other very processed items

•Candy, cookies, ice cream and various other sweets

•Whole milk and high-fat cheeses

•Natural is actually heart healthful

Just an extremely little quantity of the daily sodium intake of ours is from the saltshaker on the table and food in the natural state has little salt; it is prepared food that is the main enabler of our salt addiction. The unfortunate truth is the fact that the more we "mess around" with the food of ours filling it with ingredients, wrapping it in plastic material and typically which makes it unrecognizable from its original condition, the less great for us it becomes. This's why it's essential to eat natural foods that are whole whenever possible.

For instance, the DASH Diet emphasizes the potassium content of foods that are whole, particularly that of vegetables and fruits which helps maintain blood pressure ranges healthful. Several dairy products and fish are abundant sources of healthy potassium.

Nevertheless, vegetables and fruits are loaded with a certain type of potassium which positively influences acid base metabolism. It's thought this type of potassium can help decrease the chance of kidney stones as well as bone loss.

While you may believe that canned veggies are a healthful replacement for new ones, the opposite is usually true: canned veggies are usually laden with preservatives and frequently include extra salt. A single serving of refined cream style corn for instance, might include almost as 730 mg of sodium per cup. Select low-sodium canned frozen vegetables or vegetables with no sauces instead and consume as much fresh produce as is possible.

It can be hard to part with older favorites and lots of individuals are tempted to eat unhealthful products rather compared to waste them. Remember, although, that all these nuts are eventually going to wind up as misuse whether they undergo the body of yours or not. Exactly why should eat them when you can create healthful choices instead?

In case the budget demands of yours that you gradually phase out different things, do so and observe your food portions carefully. If you are considering keeping certain items on hand because they're family favorites, keep in your mind that what is not ideal for your personal diet is not the best for your family members' also. It may have a bit of effort to find and make replacements, though the payoff in regards to your as well as your loved ones' overall health is well worth the effort.

Then, think about where and when you usually eat unhealthful food items. In case you've an inclination to get to work vending machine if you are starving, bored and stressed at your workplace, plant a number of healthy snacks within easy access of the desk of yours. Packages of unsalted or maybe lightly salted peanuts, dried fruit and even certain power bars or perhaps meal replacement bars are able to avoid a binge.

Canned soups and also jarred pasta sauces are possible, though they usually have very high amounts of salt and extra sugar. For instance, one glass of refined chicken noodle soup generally has approximately 744 mg of salt, while a serving of condensed tomato soup has approximately 480 mg of salt and twelve grams of sugars.

Some food producers are working hard to offer their customers with better options, so look for reduced-sugar varieties and low-sodium.

Perhaps you regularly grab quick lunches out or stop by your favorite fast food joint while managing chores. To change this undesirable habit, store a few healthful snacks in the glove compartment of yours so you've an item to reach for when hunger strikes. In case particular fast food sign is bring about for unhealthful cravings, bring a unique route which will limit contact with temptation.

Gain Portion Control Awareness

Lots of individuals are surprised when they understand how much larger today's meal sizes are than they had been merely 20 years ago. It is not the fault of yours that you're eating larger portions; you've been taught to expect them. During the 1990s, the dimensions of the common dinner plate increased from ten to twelve inches across; at exactly the same period, bowls and cups likewise expanded.

That is not all; areas at restaurants are becoming massively oversized too. In reality, existing meal sizes at fast-food chains are, on typical, 2 to 5 times bigger than they had been when those restaurants had been initially established. McDonald's very first hamburger weighed in at a sensible 1.6 ounce. Nowadays, you are able to get yourself a Double Quarter Pounder with cheese which includes 2 beef patties weighing four ounce a piece before food preparation that is half a pound of beef! This monstrous sandwich has 750 calories, forty three grams of fat and also 1,280 mg of salt.

This's only one example; selection products at some other restaurants have ballooned to an outrageous size too. The best part is the fact that in case you are preparing to consume at a restaurant or even enjoy a snack from home, you are able to typically find solid info concerning calorie count, sodium online and fat. Numerous states today require restaurants to showcase calorie info on menu. Knowing what's hiding in the food of yours can be extremely helpful when it comes time to determine what to consume and what you should leave behind.

Transitioning to the DASH Diet

The choice to have a new diet program is tough, one that is going to require hard work and discipline. After you commit to incorporating the DASH Diet into the lifestyle of yours, it's crucial to successfully get ready for your journey towards wellness.

Here are a few tips and steps that you need to incorporate into the lifestyle a minimum of seven days before you formally start the DASH Diet plan.

Fresh House

Changing the eating habits of yours is a difficult task, therefore, it is better to remove temptations that might jeopardize your health. One of the greatest things you are able to do to attain success is eliminating all the off limits food in the building.

Get rid of processed foods (prepared snack food items, potato chips, foods that are fried etc.) and also high sodium and high fat condiments such as salad dressings, soybean sauces etc. You understand your very own weaknesses much better compared to anybody, so even in case food is permitted on the DASH Diet foods list, eliminate it when you yourself realize it's something you are going to have a tough time consuming in small amounts.

Plan Your Menu in Advance

The secret to become successful with the DASH Diet is always to prepare the meals of yours ahead of time. Whether you make use of the menu plans offered in the book or even make your own, it helps you to know in advance what you will be eating the first few weeks. Preparation of meal plans helps with going shopping, prepares you for a completely new method of eating and also removes unhealthy snacking once you start the diet.

Prepare Your Taste Buds

The week before you begin the diet of yours, begin to scale back on portion sizes, walk up the saltshaker from the table, choose fresh fruit with regards to dessert and bypass the unhealthy foods. Focus on these first steps and never have to be concerned about calories or perhaps any of the other facets of the DASH Diet. By the time you begin the diet of yours, the body will currently have the procedure for adjusting to the new method of taking (and intense cravings has diminished).

Begin your fitness program a week early or maybe a week late

Starting a brand new diet along with a new exercise plan at the very same time could be frustrating. In case you thrive on that type of major change, then be sure get it done. In case not, begin your fitness program the week before or maybe the week after you begin the DASH Diet. Cooking for the DASH Diet isn't about results; the thing is making the change as simple it can be. One week will not make a major impact on the health plan of yours, though it may be the difference between frustration and motivation.

The top ten tips to prepare for achievement one.

1.Trade your saltshaker for salt substitute

Plan ahead and also eliminate salt any time you are able to, so you are able to receive it in foods that are other in which it can't be eliminated. This's particularly crucial in case you've hypertension and need to stay within probably the lowest sodium edition of the diet. When possible, use another herb or salt substitutes blend rather than salt.

2.Make the correct choices the simplest ones

Make certain that fresh fruit along with other healthy snacks are definitely more noticeable than tempting treats like as chocolate that is dark and sorbet. To ward off temptation, keep snacks that are healthy and a water container accessible and stay away from the fast food lunch capture by bringing your very own foods to work.

3.Exercise first point in the morning

Something frequently gets in the form of training, particularly when a new exercise regime is now being initiated. Until you are totally hooked on fitness and not likely to work with any excuse coming the way of yours, it's ideal to exercise when you awake. It's usually easy to alter the workout schedule but hold back until working away has turned into a habit. (that usually takes approximately 30 days.)

4.Drink a ton of water

Many experts suggest drinking at least 60 4 ounces of water each day. In case you are not currently doing this, you have to start. The new diet of yours is heavy with food items which aid digestion, though you want a great deal of water getting things going. Ample water will also enable you to lose extra saved clean water, feel fuller longer and have much more energy.

5.Skip the places for the very first 2 weeks

While you should not rob yourself of things you like, like heading out to eat, it is advisable to hold back until you are accustomed to make better choices, plus seeing results that inspire you to stay with the diet plan. In case you head out to eat before the healthy choices of yours start to be second nature, you might unintentionally sabotage yourself. One breadbasket will not set you too physically, though it may do harm to the resolve of yours. Most dieters are acquainted with the anger and frustration which follows a binge or perhaps a misstep. You have to feel great about yourself and the progress of yours, therefore limit opportunities that place you off course.

6.Buddy up or get the friends of yours to help you

In case possible, enlist a relative or maybe friend to begin the diet along with you. Getting somebody to join you for training may in addition be a huge help. Accountability and also mutual motivation is a crucial element in following the plan of yours. In case you do not have any person that wishes to diet or even exercise with you, at least let the friends of yours and family understand how important your goals are to you, plus do not hesitate to question them to help take out temptation and also keep you on book.

7.Enjoy eating

The menu plans and dishes in this particular book are resources to guide you and enable you to stick to the DASH Diet. They're not, nonetheless, ready in stone. Feel free to design your very own menu programs with the meals list, your day serving's guide, along with the thousands of DASH friendly dishes available. If you are not enjoying the food of yours, you will not be on the diet regime for very long.

8.Keep a journal

Have a small notebook available and jot down your progress. Write down what you consume and just how you feel; after consuming a healthy meal, a great workout or winning a fight against temptation. These notes may actually help keep you inspired, particularly when you reach a rough patch.

9.Stay away from or plan for meals triggers

Almost all individuals have specific triggers that cause overeating or making terrible food choices. Determine the triggers of yours and discover ways to stay away from them entirely or at minimum to outwit them. In case watching TV is not the same without any snacks, then have an abundance of good ones on hand or even eliminate TV for the very first few weeks. Bad habits are a lot easier to stay away from once the habit inducing trigger is recognized.

10.Take action!

Chapter 6 What Should You Eat? What Shouldn't You Eat? The Do's and the Don'ts

Food this is one of the most loved topics. At the mention of food, most people smile because food is lovable - it causes excitement in the mind and to the body. Food is a basic necessity in life, something you can't leave without, something that should be done at least thrice in a day. That is a lot of topics to be discussed at the mention of food based on certain principles. Be it healthy, fitness, sweetness, or worst. This section will be focusing on the do's and don'ts of food, what to eat, and what not to eat.

What to Eat

Everyone loves food, like really a lot won't even complete a conversation with the mention of food. Especially those who love cooking, the food is everything. When it comes to what to eat, the topic is ambiguous, unless it is explained into small topics. The discussion is hard to break. The following are some of the major considerations that need to be observed considering what food to eat.

1.   Health

2.   Weight

3.   Bodybuilding

4.   Time

5.   Disease Medication

6.   Situation (pregnancy)

Every food has a purpose, people eat with different reasons and purpose objective.

Eating healthy

Eating healthy is very important, that is making sure that you are eating a balanced diet. That involves grains, vegetables, fruits, proteins, and foods rich in low fats. A person eating healthy is a person watching out for his/her body, someone who actually cares about how people view his/her body. This is a person who wants to look and feel good about the body. Healthy eating is eating food that is given prescription by the doctor. This is the foods that don't have excessive proteins or excessive calories but are all of the equal measures.

Healthy foods are categorized under different groups; the fats, proteins, carbohydrates, and fiber. Together in portions, they make a healthy result. Below is a list of some of the foods to be eaten in these categories and the portions to be taken in order to stay healthy.

Fats

This is foods that are rich in calories and should be definitely watched out for so as not to be eaten in excess. If the fats are eaten in excess, the result will be definitely obesity. Furthermore, obesity is not just bad but dangerous. It is a motivation of a lot of diseases.

Some examples of fats foods include:

☐ Biscuits

☐ Cakes

☐ Fried foods

☐ Butter and margarine in bread

Fats in most cases are advised to be eaten in small portions for body safety.

Proteins

Proteins are the other food category that is highly valued in the body as they do most of the inner activities of the body like the regulation of both body and organ's tissue. Proteins are the source of food that should be dominating the most on the menu. They help in the development of bones and muscles in the body which are used in a lot of activities in everyday life. Most of the proteins are found in animal products.

Four reasons why you should put protein in your menu:

a) They are involved in repairing body tissues.

b) They help in fighting the body through diseases by the white blood cell.

c) They are involved in most transportation that takes place in the body.

d) The right amount of protein in the body is an assurance of the right growth and development of the baby or child and even for pregnant women.

Proteins are generally classified under four categories of structures.

• Primary structure

• Secondary structure

• Tertiary structure

- Quaternary structure

The four structures are determined by the DNA and RNA that are found in the body.

Examples of protein foods include the following:

☐ Baked beans

☐ Chapatti

☐ Meat

☐ Fish

☐ Eggs

☐ Cereal milk

☐ Legumes

☐ Red meat

Carbohydrates

This is food rich in molecules that are made up of three major sources: carbon, hydrogen, and oxygen. In some cases, they are also referred to as starchy foods.

Examples of carbohydrates include the following:

☐ Bread

☐ Rice both white and brown

☐ Potatoes

Fiber

Fiber foods are also very important in this category and are eaten in great portions. This is a category of food that is prescribed by the doctor in great portion to be eaten in plenty. According to the current research that is observed in many situations, fiber comes with a lot of benefits. Like for instance, it prevents the body from filling empty and keeps it fuller most of the times. Apart from that, fiber is well known to reduce the chances of diabetes in the body as well as lowers the amount of cholesterol found in the body.

Examples of fiber include the following:

☐ Fruits

☐ Vegetables

- ☐ Whole grain breakfast

- ☐ Nuts

- ☐ Brown rice

The best tip of increasing fiber in fruits is by not peeling the skin off but instead wash it well and eat it as a whole.

Why eat healthily

Some people just eat healthy because it is recommended by the doctor but not because they know the importance of sticking to healthy foods.

Below are some of the reasons why you should eat healthily.

- ☐ Keeps you in good weight

- ☐ Makes you feel good about yourself

- ☐ Reduce diseases

Weight

Your body size determines a lot what you should or should not eat at all. A person trying to gain weight and a person trying to lose weight will definitely eat something very different at the end of the day. The one trying to increase weight will eat a lot of foods rich in calories, while the one trying to lose weight will make sure to reduce foods rich in calories in the menu and rather go for the vegetables.

What not to eat when trying to lose weight

- Sugary drinks

- Candy bars

- Ice cream

- Fried foods

- Cream in milk

Those are some of the foods that you should definitely watch out for and be very serious when it comes to them. If you dare try them out, you will be gaining more fat than losing weight. They may seem less harmful when you see them because they are very sweet but in reality, they motivate a lot in gearing up the calories in the body. Instead of them, I would recommend you go for less harmful types with less or zero calories in them. Try out the following list to your menu and within a month, there will be an impeccable change in your body.

- Lean meat, chicken breast

- Smashed potatoes

- Brown rice

- Green peas

- Pork Fillet

The above will not only help you reduce weight but keep you in very good shape.

According to the health station, for any change to be observed effective when it comes to losing weight, exercise is needed to boost up the changes and speed the process. For beginners, it is important not to just look for a proper diet as a method of losing weight, but also exercise as a method of speeding up the process.

These exercises can be indoors or outdoors. Some of the outdoors activities include running, swimming, hiking, and housework activities at the compound of the house. The indoors activates include squats, push-ups, press ups, weightlifting, and treadmill.

Importance of exercise for weight loss

a) Prevent diseases

There are so many diseases that come with obesity and some of them can be prevented by proper and regular exercises if done in the right way. Exercise helps to prevent heart diseases with activities like swimming. The exercises are important in burning up calories in the body, it helps to keep the body in balance especially with activities like hiking, and exercise sets the mood of a person and therefore ending up in reducing stress and depressions that may have occurred. Most of the overweight people suffer from swollen knees, therefore with the help of running exercise, improvement on the knees will definitely be seen.

b) Keeps the body fit

It is through these activities that the body is able to achieve balance by its own. Exercise makes people regain proper weight that is prescribed by the doctor and keeps them in the right shape. House chores are very important in initiating changes in the overweight as it requires efforts to move and pull things from one place to another. Exercises most of the time end up giving this person more muscles and fewer fats at the end of the day, if done well.

At times, people go to the gym and still not see any changes in their body because of not adhering to simple rules like:

a) Lifting the very lightweight

b) The wrong plan meal

c) Wasting a lot of time in the gym doing other things rather than workout

d) Doing the lifts the wrong way

e) Being lazy and going to the gym twice a week instead of twice a day

f) Not change your workout routine and doing it every day

As you can see, it is evident in this section that people at this level are not eating because they are hungry but instead they are eating because they want to reduce weight and keep in shape like other people. Overweight is one of the most dangerous encounters to ever have, it may even lead to death as it is well known to contribute to most of cancers diseases.

Bodybuilding

Foods that are rich in the development of bones and muscles, in most cases, they are proteins. This is the people who eat food because they want to increase mass in their body and become big. Proteins are therefore that kind of luxury, but again, be careful of the calories, you might overdo them and end up fat instead of fit. Some people might be tempted to try out calories and proteins because they speed up the process but they ought to know that it will always lead to being fat rather than fit because calories are known to dominate in most cases when misused.

Bodybuilding foods are mostly preferred by those doing jobs or work that require a lot of efforts like those that are working in constructions or queries. These people use a lot of efforts that drains their energy at the end of the day. Foods rich in proteins are more proper for them.

Time

Time is very essential when it comes to eating. Like the scriptures say, there is time for everything and everything should be done at the right time and not just randomly because it is supposed to be done.

What to eat is controlled by time under three distinctions: the breakfast, lunch, and supper. Every of this time has something that is recommended and according to the nutritionist, what you can eat at lunchtime is not what you should eat in the morning, everything with its own time. To some people, eating breakfast is not a must, they would prefer skipping it and eating heavy lunch instead. Well, there is no harm to that but the truth is all the three types of meals are very important and none should be skipped at all.

What to have for breakfast

This is one of the meals that have a history of being eaten in the wrong way. Most people don't know the proper meal plan for breakfast because they are not used to eat. Well, do not worry, I got your back on that. Below are some right choices preferred for breakfast in the morning.

• Eggs - according to most research, eggs is one of the most preferred meals in the morning and is used to help reduce blood sugar in the body especially the egg yolk.

• Greek yogurt - yogurt is rich in proteins and provides energy in the body. Yogurt is mostly preferred because they keep the stomach full for long before they feel empty again.

• Coffee - those who do or spent a lot of times in the office prefer coffee to tea mainly because coffee is well known to ensure that the body remains alert and the mood is often jovial.

• Nuts - nuts are not only sweet and tasty in nature, but they are also very important when it comes to monitoring the body weight to ensure you don't get fat to obesity.

What to have for lunch

Some say breakfast is more important than lunch, some argue that the vice versa is true. Well, personally, don't let anyone fool you otherwise. Lunch is a very important part of the meal and is there mainly to help you get through the afternoon with a full stomach. Lunch is more effective especially when it is taken in the right way and in the right proportion. Below are some of the best options to consider for your lunchtime hour.

• Vegetables

• Sandwich

• Chicken salad

• Chips

• Black beans

• Potatoes

Lunch is important in various ways. For instance, lunch is important because it helps to increase the blood sugar during the day which results in concentration and alertness for the rest of the afternoon. Skipping lunch for those who take it likely should know that is very wrong and comes with severe consequences especially when you are working or a student. This is because when you skip lunch, chances of distractions and lots of attention in classes are very high which leads to poor performance at the end of the day.

What to have for supper

Supper is one of the hectic times in the meal plan and most people find it hard to stick to, especially the bachelors living alone. This is the people who leave for work early and return to the house late at night with tired bodies and mind. At this point, the mind is mostly tired and it just wants you to go to the shower, take a warm clean bath, and go to sleep till the next day. That occurs in a lot of times to most workers especially the low wage workers who are underpaid and work the most hours. Below are some simple foods you can prepare for your supper that get cooked and are ready within a short time.

• Spaghetti

- Beef stew

- Tuna and avocado

- Chicken bake

- scrambled eggs

- Broccoli

Those are some of the quickest foods to prepare for your supper within a short time before going to bed or if not in a hurry, you can try brown rice, fried meat, or fish.

Disease curing

Some people eat food for curing diseases as the main purpose at the end of the day. It is so true that these foods are not like the rest. I don't mean they taste different, but I mean they are situated in a very strict meal that ought to be followed under all situations in order to go well with the medicine provided by the doctor.

Fruits are mostly preferred in these situations especially the banana that helps in controlling the blood sugar level in the body. Yogurt is used to pushing medicine faster to the expected area, vegetable green foods like kales and spinach help to maintain the body and prevent weight gain at any time.

Situation

Some foods are taken based on certain situations and many of this time there is never otherwise of any alternative. It might be a prison form of situation, where you have to eat what other people are eating and there is no other option of selection, or it might be a pregnancy situation where a mother has to eat right in order to deliver a healthy baby when due.

Having known what to eat and when to eat and why to eat, we will then focus on the don'ts of what not to eat and the worst foods never to try in your menu as a concluding part.

What Not to Eat

☐ Microwave foods

The microwave is good for most people because they are fast to cook and save a lot of time to people especially those that prefer preparing quick foods. Well, that is good. It really helps a lot, but at the same time, the microwave is known to come with severe issues too. Like for instance, it may lead to diabetes or the fact that the food prepared is never evenly cooked.

☐ Hot dogs

It is true that they are very sweet and tasty and most people prefer buying them during sports activities or after running in the street. Hot dogs are junk foods and are rich in fats that lead to overweight if proper actions are not taken. The major danger that comes with it is the presence of sodium in them which is not needed in the body at all.

☐   Doughnuts

Doughnuts are the other sweet type of cakes that are loved by a lot of people because of their tasty allure. The sad truth is that these doughnuts are prepared by the GMO's which often leads to cancer when taken in excess and can even cause fast death from clogging the arteries.

☐   Pizza

What is the first thing that comes to mind when you think of pizza? I don't know about you, but my first is that it is yummy. Pizza is the top in the list of the world eaten junk food with the most deliveries in a day. Most people love to order pizza during house parties or when left alone in the house by the parents or when there is no food in the house to eat and you are desperate for food in the stomach. Pizza is mixed with a lot of things that are rich in calories and that is the major reason why you should stop eating pizza from today.

Chapter 7 Advantages And Disadvantages Of The Dash Diet

The DASH diet (Dietary Approaches to Stop Hypertension) has been reliably referred to as extraordinary compared to other by and large diets. The deep-rooted eating plan centers around devouring natural products, vegetables, lean proteins, and entire grains.1 Foods that are high in sodium or included sugar are diminished.

The DASH program was created by a board of specialists at the National Institutes of Health to assist Americans with bringing down their blood pressure.2 But for reasons unknown, it can likewise advance solid weight reduction and may give other medical advantages, also.

Notwithstanding, there is no eating routine that is ideal for everybody. Consider the upsides and downsides of this eating plan before you start the eating routine.

Stars

Proof based medical advantages

Available

Adaptable

Wholesome parity

Intended for long lasting wellbeing

Sponsored by significant wellbeing associations

Cons

Difficult to keep up

Costly

No accommodation nourishments

No composed help

Requires significant nourishment following

Not intended for weight reduction

May not be proper for everybody

Experts

Proof Based Health Benefits

The DASH diet has been considered widely. The first investigation which presented the eating plan was distributed in 1997 and indicated that the eating regimen decreased hypertension in individuals with ordinary circulatory strain and diminished it much more in those with hypertension.

Since that unique investigation was presented, later research has affirmed the discoveries. Indeed, creators of a 2016 investigation reasoned that "the DASH dietary methodology may be the best dietary measure to lessen circulatory strain among hypertensive and pre-hypertensive patients dependent on top notch proof."

What's more, the individuals who pursue the eating plan can expect other medical advantages. Further research has discovered that the DASH diet diminishes LDL cholesterol, and may improve other cardiovascular hazard factors, too. The DASH diet has been demonstrated to be a compelling administration technique for diabetes and research has even indicated that the DASH diet may decrease the danger of gout in men.

Notwithstanding examines supporting the DASH diet explicitly, look into has reliably discovered that decreasing your sugar admission, disposing of intensely handled, sodium-rich nourishments, and expanding your admission of foods grown from the ground prompts a wide scope of wellbeing benefits.

Open

The nourishment suggested on the DASH diet can be effectively found in practically any general store. There are no elusive fixings, required nourishments, enhancements, or memberships required to pursue the program.

Also, not at all like business diet plans, all that you have to become familiar with the program is accessible online for nothing out of pocket. The National Institutes of Health gives a wide scope of assets, including a total manual for prescribed servings, dinner plans, sodium consumption suggestions, calorie guides, tip sheets, and plans.

There are likewise endless cookbooks, sites, and cell phone applications devoted to this eating style. What's more, since it has been all around explored and broadly advanced in the therapeutic community4 , this is an eating routine that your social insurance supplier is probably going to be acquainted with. Along these lines, in the event that you have inquiries regarding whether to pursue the arrangement, they might be well-prepared to give counsel.

Adaptable

Run diet plans are accessible for different calorie levels to suit people with various action levels.1 It is anything but difficult to decide the correct vitality consumption dependent on the online graphs gave by NIH.

Also, the individuals who pursue unique weight control plans can pursue the DASH eating plan. Veggie lovers and vegans5 will discover the arrangement simple to pursue since grains, organic products, and vegetables are emphatically empowered. The individuals who eat a sans gluten diet can keep up their eating program by picking safe grains, for example, buckwheat and quinoa. Furthermore, the individuals who eat a genuine or Halal eating routine can pick nourishments that comply with those dietary principles and still pursue the arrangement.

Nourishing Balance

While numerous weight control plans expect buyers to definitely move their macronutrient balance (counting low-carb diets or low-fat eating regimens) or seriously limit calories, the DASH diet remains inside dietary rules gave by the USDA.

For instance, on the DASH diet, you'll expend about 55% of your calories from carbohydrate.6 The USDA prescribes that 45% to 65% of your calories originate from carbs.

As indicated by the USDA, 20% to 35% of your calories should originate from fat and under 10% of those calories ought to be immersed fat. On the DASH diet, close to 27% of your calories will originate from fat and up to six percent of those calories will be soaked fat.

By following the program, you ought to likewise have the option to arrive at your prescribed admission of other significant supplements, for example, protein, fiber, and calcium.

Long lasting Wellness

The DASH diet is certainly not a momentary program. The eating plan is intended to be a way of life that you keep up for life.

Tips are given to enable the individuals who to expend a run of the mill American eating routine slowly acclimate to eating less red meat, less handled nourishments, and more foods grown from the ground. Changes are acquainted step by step with advance adherence.

For instance, DASH specialists suggest that you slice your sodium admission to 2,300 milligrams for each day before endeavoring to decrease it to 1,500 milligrams1 — a level that may give more noteworthy medical advantages to a few. Moreover, there is no troublesome early on stage where calories or day by day carbs are definitely cut.

Sponsored By Major Health Organizations

The DASH diet has been advanced by the National Institutes of Health, National Heart, Lung, and Blood Institute, the American Heart Association, the American Diabetes Association, the USDA and restorative establishments including the Mayo Clinic and the Cleveland Clinic. The DASH diet is likewise positioned as the second-best diet generally by U.S. News and World Report.

Cons

Difficult to Maintain

The individuals who eat a run of the mill American eating routine may make some hard memories acclimating to the DASH plan. The program suggests that you slice your salt admission to 2,300 milligrams of sodium for each day and possibly to 1,500 milligrams for every day.

As indicated by the Centers for Disease Control, the normal American devours 3,400 milligrams of sodium for every day. Quite a bit of our salt admission originates from vigorously prepared nourishments—which are confined on the DASH diet.

What's more, regardless of whether you don't eat handled nourishments, relinquishing the salt-shaker propensity is hard for many.

Therefore and for a few others, the DASH diet can be trying to adhere to. An examination exploring DASH diet consistence found that individuals make some hard memories adhering to the program and need something other than guiding to stay with it as long as possible.

Analysts have additionally examined the dietary fat admission on the DASH diet, guessing that permitting increasingly fat in the eating routine may assist individuals with staying with the arrangement.

In one examination, members pursued a higher fat form of the eating routine and expended full-fat dairy items rather than low-fat or nonfat dairy and furthermore decreased their sugar admission by restricting utilization of organic product juice. Scientists found that the higher fat form of the DASH diet brought circulatory strain down to a similar degree as the customary DASH diet without fundamentally expanding LDL cholesterol.

Costly

One of the most regularly refered to worries about the DASH diet is that it tends to be costly.

Crisp products of the soil are progressively costly as well as they turn sour quicker which may prompt nourishment waste. Canned and solidified nourishments are frequently less expensive however may contain included sugars or sodium. Crisp meat and fish can likewise be pricey.

Nonetheless, with savvy arranging and practice, this "con" can transform into a "genius." Planning ahead, making supper plans, acquiring occasional produce, and purchasing in mass are generally brilliant approaches to decrease nourishment costs. These are likewise brilliant practices that advance good dieting and can assist you with sticking to the DASH diet.

Since the DASH is certainly not a business diet, you won't have the option to get pre-bundled nourishments conveyed to your entryway. You additionally can't go to the cooler area of your neighborhood showcase and get dinners that are as of now cooked. There are no simple to-get smoothies or lunch rooms. This eating routine takes more work.

No Organized Support

Another well-known component of some eating routine plans is bunch support. A few projects offer vis-à-vis guiding, bunch gatherings, or distributed instructing. These highlights assist individuals with overcoming unpleasant patches when inspiration fades, enables them to pose inquiries, and learn shrewd tips and insider tricks.

While you'll discover a lot of DASH diet assets accessible, there is no sorted out help stage for the arrangement. Notwithstanding, on the off chance that you are thinking about the eating program, don't let this "con" wreck you. Any great enrolled dietitian knows about the arrangement and they can assist you with developing supper designs, or give instructing and bolster when you need it.

Requires Food Tracking

There is no calorie checking required on the DASH diet. In any case, there are suggested calorie objectives that decide the quantity of servings you are considered every nutrition class. So you'll need to pick the correct level and modify occasionally as your age changes or on the off chance that you increment or reduction your action level. All things considered, you don't need to track or check calories.

Be that as it may, to pursue the DASH diet appropriately, you have to quantify parts and check servings of nourishments that fall into various categories. This procedure can be similarly as dreary, if not more along these lines, than calorie tallying.

The DASH diet control gave by the National Institutes of Health incorporates a few downloadable structures that can be printed out to assist you with overseeing and track your servings of food.17 With training, the procedure may get simpler. Yet, at first, this piece of the program might be overpowering for certain individuals.

Not Specifically Designed for Weight Loss

While you can pursue a lower-calorie target plan on the DASH diet, the essential accentuation isn't on weight reduction. Moreover, thinks about researching the DASH diet don't concentrate on weight reduction, yet rather on other wellbeing outcomes.4 So it tends to be difficult to advise how the DASH diet looks at to different eating regimens when you're attempting to get in shape.

The DASH diet does exclude a brisk weight reduction stage (offered by numerous other health improvement plans) in which shoppers can thin down rapidly to help inspiration and adherence to the arrangement. Rather, you are probably going to see steady weight loss.

Not Appropriate for Everyone

While there are numerous individuals who can profit by the DASH diet, analysts have recognized certain gatherings who should practice alert before changing their dietary patterns to embrace this arrangement.

A distributed report explored the DASH diet in exceptional populaces. While study creators note that the eating regimen is solid for the vast majority, they exhort that patients with incessant kidney sickness, ceaseless liver infection, and the individuals who are recommended renin-angiotensin-aldosterone framework foe should practice alert. They additionally recommend that changes to the DASH diet might be essential for patients with ceaseless cardiovascular breakdown, uncontrolled diabetes mellitus type II, lactose narrow mindedness, and celiac disease.

The report underscores the significance of cooperating with your human services supplier before rolling out considerable improvements to your eating routine or exercise program. They cannot just give direction with respect to the potential medical advantages you may pick up, yet they might have the option to allude you to an enlisted dietitian or another expert who can offer help and related administrations.

Chapter 8 Myths about the DASH Diet

As with any popular eating plan, there are often (at the least) misconceptions and (to the extreme) conspiracy theories. While thin-foil hatters and flat Earthers haven't really found time for the DASH diet, there have been some erroneous notions about the side effects of following this eating plan and what should or should not be done on the diet.

Since this book, DASH Diet, thrives on facts, we cannot allow these myths persist.

This chapter isn't to make anyone feel dumb for what they have previously believed about DASH. Instead, we will be debunking certain myths in order to make you less afraid to give DASH a try. This eating plan could very well lead to the most positive life changes you have yet experienced.

Ready? Then let's go!

1.   5-9 daily servings of fruits and vegetables is impossible: One reason many people get this wrong is because they don't really get what a serving is. If you also think that no one can or should eat 5-9 daily servings of fruits and veggies, then you likely imagine a serving to be as large as a single watermelon.

In fact, one small banana equals one serving. How impossible is it to eat a few bananas in a day. The next day, you could have half of an avocado. That's also a single serving. Five halves (servings) of avocado amounts to two and a half avocados. Not that big a deal, right.

2.   You want to eat healthy, but fruits and vegetables are too expensive: This is an offshoot of the argument that healthy foods are more costly to purchase than junk or unhealthy food.

But it isn't exactly true. You hear people talk about how it is becoming increasingly cheaper to just buy meals to-go, than cook them from scratch at home. This opinion is often expressed by people who may or may not be money rich, but are definitely time poor. Coming home from work, the last thing on the minds of such people is cooking. People may also assume that surviving on fruits and veggies is not exactly as filling as a greasy burrito or cheeseburger. As such, many think that to feel the same level of satisfaction, they would eat even more apples or cucumbers and spend much more money. As you read through the recipes later in the book, you'll see how easy (and cheap) it can be to get your servings in without breaking the bank.

Concrete studies have shown that half a cup of fruits and veggies (one serving) costs about 40 cents. So, whether you want to have five or nine servings of fruits and vegetables, you will most likely be spending no more than $3-4

3.   You just can't make fruits and vegetables taste good: How pleasantly shocked you will be after reading this book!

People honestly try with their vegetables and fruits. They purchase the canned produce, but whatever deliciousness might exist just doesn't seem to register on their taste buds. Fresh fruits take way too long to prepare for an individual who is quite hangry. How about frozen vegetables? Someone might tell you they become complete duds after being cooked. They are wrong.

There are ways to go about preparing finger-licking meals with fruits and vegetables. It will, of course, require your willingness to learn and try out new things. If you try the recipes to be shared later on in this book, you will find your mindset changed.

4.   Freezing or canning makes fruits and vegetables less nutritious: This is one that most of us have heard since we were little children. Apparently, fruits and vegetables are only good when they are fresh.

It might interest you to know that not only are the nutrients lost by canning or freezing minimal to the point of being negligible, a greater portion of the nutrients are preserved better than fresh fruits and vegetables. The lost nutrients are so small because canned produce undergoes processing a short while after harvesting. That means, canned and frozen veggies or fruits are packaged when they reach peak freshness.

They are processed to have a long shelf life (canned produce more than the frozen ones). And this means that they will outlast your fresh plant produce. Since frozen and canned produce are more economical than their fresh counterparts, you may want to choose them once in a while.

5.   To up your vitamin C intake, your best bet is citrus: This is why many folks think of oranges when vitamin C is mentioned. Oranges, tangerines, and other citrus fruits are great, but bell peppers pack more vitamin C than those fruits. A tennis ball sized bell pepper has a vitamin C content as high as 300 mg. That's a hundred times more than an orange of the same size.

You have the freedom to think broadly as you try to meet your daily recommended intake of vitamin C. Among your list of choices are kiwis, pineapples, strawberries, broccoli, cantaloupes, grapefruits, tangerines, and brussels sprouts.

6.   You can have as much vitamin C as you want: Of course, you can. But you absolutely should not. vitamin C is easily and quickly removed from the body. While you should have a lot of it daily, there is a limit.

To exceed 2000 mg in one day is playing dangerously close to the edge. Many people go over this dosage and don't report any side effects, but there is the possibility of suffering heartburn, vomiting, diarrhea, insomnia, and kidney stones.

It's best to avoid such risks. The point is to be healthy and not place yourself unnecessarily in harm's way.

7.   Fiber exists in just one form: You now know about soluble and insoluble fibers. You also know that different foods provide various kinds of fiber. For example, while insoluble fibers can be gotten from wheat bran, flaxseeds provide soluble fiber.

And these different types of dietary fibers perform different functions in the body. If you need a refresher on the functions of dietary fiber. The point here is that fiber isn't fiber, even though both kinds are awesome.

8.   Drinking fruit juice on the DASH diet is a big no-no: This, while definitely a myth, bears some resemblance to the truth. But only so much.

The trick here (which really isn't a trick) is to only go for fruit juice labeled 100% juice. If that's the case, then all you're really missing out on is the fiber. If it is labeled 100% juice, it implies that there are no added sugars or even water. Not only do 100% juice drinks taste way better, they provide you with all the nutrients you would have gotten from a fresh fruit.

As an adult, try not to exceed 4-8 oz of fruit juice every day. This should amount to 1-2 servings.

9.   You can have as much fiber as you want: The rule stands that too much of anything is a potential health hazard. Whether it is water, vitamin C, or fiber, moderation is key.

Just because fiber is such a good nutrient for you doesn't mean it won't cause you abdominal pain, diarrhea, or IBS (Irritable Bowel Syndrome) when you abuse it. This is especially the case with insoluble fiber. But, it is pretty rare that an individual consumes fiber to the point that they experience such side effects.

Just in case, the daily recommended limit of dietary fiber for men is 38 g. For women, it's 25 g.

10.   You can't follow the DASH diet because you're genetically inclined to crave salt: Some folks believe that cutting down the amount of salt they consume will be harder for them than for others, because their love for sodium is DNA deep.

Well, good news! Your perceived inability to stop eating that much salt is not a natural craving. It's just something you've trained your body to want. As such, you can always retrain yourself to consume less sodium before it leads to serious health issues. There is no better time to start than with your next meal.

Carefully seek out labels like Salt Reduced, No Added Salt, Low Salt, or Zero Salt on whatever packaged good you want to purchase. Also, be mindful about the amount of salt you add to what you cook.

11.   Taking more vitamin C will cure your cold: This is one myth that many experts in the field of nutrition presently enjoy shooting down. So, you've probably heard or read it somewhere before. But did you know how this myth began?

In a really weird twist, one of the greatest minds in history gave birth to this misconception. His name was Linus Pauling, and you may have heard of him if you studied molecular biology in college. Pauling received two Nobel prizes and is credited with revealing the true nature of chemical bonds and discovering that sickle cell anemia, is in fact, a disease at a molecular level.

A great mind indeed. How then is this genius of a man the source of something so unscientific, yet compelling enough to mislead people so many years after?

The part of the myth being compelling is understandable, since Pauling had won his Nobel in Peace and Chemistry before coming up with the vitamin C myth. So when he published his book, Vitamin C and The Common Cold, America, and the rest of the world after, lapped it all up. Fifty years after the publication of that book, and the myth still persists.

He made, quite frankly, outlandish claims that vitamin C in high doses (as much as 3000 mg) was, in effect, a cure-all. The common cold was the least of all the illnesses Linus Pauling claimed could be cured or prevented by taking lots of vitamin C. Leprosy, the various kinds of cancer are but a few of all that vitamin C has the ability to cure—as purported by Pauling.

People were only too happy to ignore every other scientific organization that refuted his baseless claims and pointed out the obvious holes in his clinical trial. They were also happy to turn a blind eye when vitamin C couldn't save him from the claws of prostate cancer in 1994.

Why is it necessary to point out this particular myth in this book? It's so that you don't erroneously believe that the DASH diet will cure you of every health issue or prevent them. The fact is that vitamin C has been proven to lower blood pressure and shorten the lifespan of your common cold. That's a BIG DEAL.

No need to exaggerate the healing powers of the vitamin or endanger yourself by taking way too much Vitamin C. A high dosage of vitamin C can lead to serious health issues if you have hereditary hemochromatosis or, in simpler terms, an overload of iron (Chodosh, 2017). At the least, you might be plagued with diarrhea, which is no joke.

12.   White potatoes contain fat and should be avoided: People who have chosen to try out the DASH are often advised to run from white potatoes, and only eat sweet potatoes. This isn't just a myth, but an unnecessary one to even bother yourself with.

Whether white or sweet, if you eat a hefty amount of potatoes or fry them, you can expect that your calorie intake for the day has skyrocketed. A medium-sized potato contains about 160 calories. In that same size of potato, you have about 1000 mg of vitamin C and 4 g of fiber. Despite the number of calories contained in potatoes, they also possess so many nutrients that to avoid them, sweet or white, is really cheating yourself.

What you need to concern yourself with is the size of potato you are eating. Make them ¼ of your meals. Also, consider baked potatoes as an alternative to fried potatoes.

13.   Bananas are full of calories and should be avoided: Like white potatoes, bananas have become infamous for causing weight gain. Again, you would be short changing yourself by closing your eyes to the many nutrients packed in one medium sized banana.

As a matter of fact, there are about 105 calories in a banana of medium size. But did you know that your favorite doctor-recommended apple has nothing on that banana when it comes to vitamins A and C? Bananas, though quite low in proteins, at least have more than apples.

Another thing to note, bananas are low in fat. Most of that 105 calories (90% to be exact) are carbs. Bananas are also rich in antioxidants.

Of your recommended daily intake, a banana has 12% potassium, 20% vitamin B6, and 17% vitamin C. Bananas also contain 3.1 g of fiber which, when compared to the calories, is huge (West, 2016).

As with potatoes, you need only be conscious of what size of banana you are consuming on a daily basis. Also, you should eat fewer ripe bananas in order to promote your weight loss. Eat more unripe bananas instead, as they contain resistant starch that makes you feel satiated.

14.   Eating raw veggies will always lead to indigestion: This myth is, in fact, true (paradox much?). That is if your diet consists of raw vegetables and nothing more. If you eat raw vegetables and nothing else, then the cellulose in those raw plants will be too much work for your digestive system.

To avoid indigestion, you must compromise in either of these ways: cook those veggies or eat them alongside other foods. When you cook your raw veggies, the fiber in them can really act to aid digestion. Veggies like collards or brussels sprouts should either be fermented or cooked before they are consumed.

You can also mix the raw vegetables with fiber rich foods, and you'll be fine. Additionally, chewing your raw vegetables completely (about twenty times every time you take a bite) will make it easier for your digestive system to break them down further.

15.   If raw vegetables are not eaten cold, the nutrient is lost: Frankly speaking, this myth is probably the result of a prank gone viral. It's either that or it was started by someone who just loves cold, raw vegetables, and needed a way to justify their preference.

That's because the belief is not only unfounded, but there's no point to it. If you are not fond of cold vegetables, you can heat them. Now, this isn't the same as cooking them. You're just making them warm, and would still be eating raw vegetables.

16.   There's no point eating lettuce and celery, since they contain no nutrients: Until science proves otherwise, then foods contain nutrients if they are edible and grow from the earth. Celery and lettuce are no exception. One reason why people may have come to this conclusion is because of how much water is contained in those veggies.

Still, this isn't reason enough to ignore the many vitamins and other nutrients they have to offer. In 100 g of lettuce, there is as much as 148% of vitamin A. In addition, there is a 4% iron, 15% vitamin C, and 0% fat in the same g of lettuce.

How about celery? Eating a hundred grams of celery will provide you with 7% fiber, 6% vitamin C, 10% vitamin A, and 0% fat. So, while these veggies are mostly water—a whopping 105 g of water in celery—that should not stop you from enjoying their many nutrients.

17.   Fiber is only good to keep you regular: You probably believe that since your digestive system is working fine, there is no need to eat more fiber. In other words, keeping you regular is all fiber is good for. If you hold this as the truth, you have it wrong my friend.

There is another incentive to get a high fiber diet like DASH. It's called antioxidants. This is important because the DASH diet isn't just about losing weight.

And antioxidants are just perfect for managing heart diseases and diabetes. But that isn't the extent of fiber's benefits. Foods rich in fiber often contain prebiotics like pectin and resistant starch. While tongue savors the taste of the food you are eating, there are some bacteria in your body that act in your favor and would also like something to eat. They feed on the prebiotics and in return, your immune system receives a boost.

18.   If you need a high intake of fiber, any fruit or vegetable works fine: If the vegetable or fruit is edible and doesn't cause you any health issues, then you should include it in your diet. But don't think that all veggies and fruits contain equal amounts of fiber. The fiber content of various fruits and vegetables vary widely.

While broccoli and pears are just chock full of fibers, watermelon cannot make the same claim. This doesn't mean that watermelons aren't filled with necessary phytochemicals and antioxidants. You just won't be getting close to the same amount of fiber as you would from an avocado.

Chapter 9 21 Day Meal Plan

Days	Breakfast	Lunch	Dinner
1	Sweet Potatoes With Coconut Flakes	Veggie Quesadillas	Spinach Rolls
2	Flaxseed & Banana Smoothie	Chicken Wraps	Goat Cheese Fold-Overs
3	Fruity Tofu Smoothie	Black Bean Patties With Cilantro	Crepe Pie
4	French Toast With Applesauce	Lunch Rice Bowls	Coconut Soup
5	Banana-Peanut Butter 'N Greens Smoothie	Salmon Salad	Fish Tacos
6	Baking Powder Biscuits	Stuffed Mushrooms Caps	Cobb Salad
7	Oatmeal Banana Pancakes With Walnuts	Tuna Salad	Cheese Soup
8	Creamy Oats, Greens & Blueberry Smoothie	Shrimp Lunch Rolls	Tuna Tartare
9	Banana & Cinnamon Oatmeal	Turkey Sandwich With Mozzarella	Clam Chowder
10	Bagels Made Healthy	Veggie Soup	Asian Beef Salad
11	Cereal With Cranberry-Orange Twist	Avocado And Melon Salad	Carbonara
12	No Cook Overnight Oats	Spaghetti Squash And Sauce	Cauliflower Soup With Seeds
13	Avocado Cup With Egg	Sausage With Potatoes	Prosciutto-Wrapped Asparagus
14	Mediterranean Toast	Beef Soup	Stuffed Bell Peppers
15	Almond Butter-Banana Smoothie	Shrimp Salad	Stuffed Eggplants With Goat Cheese
16	Brown Sugar Cinnamon	Watercress, Asparagus	Korma Curry

	Oatmeal	And Shrimp Salad	
17	Buckwheat Pancakes With Vanilla Almond Milk	Chicken Tacos	Zucchini Bars
18	Tomato Bruschetta With Basil	Millet Cakes	Mushroom Soup
19	Sweet Corn Muffins	Lentils Dal With Yogurt	Stuffed Portobello Mushrooms
20	Scrambled Eggs With Mushrooms And Spinach	Lunch Quinoa And Spinach Salad	Lettuce Salad
21	Chia And Oat Breakfast Bran	Italian Pasta With Parmesan	Spinach Rolls

Chapter 10 Implementing The DASH Diet In Your Life

The DASH diet allows one to enjoy a wide variety of foods from different food groups. This approach means that there will be more nutrients in the body and the body will be able to function at an optimal level.

Instead of cutting out foods and being very restrictive with what you eat, this diet emphasizes portion control. After all, too much of a good thing can end up being harmful. We also know that some foods just naturally have more nutrients in them, and these are the foods we want to eat more of, whereas some foods have less nutrients in them and more fat or sugar, so these are the foods we want to limit.

Focusing on whole foods means that you can control what you are eating and you know what is going into your body. It is easier to control sodium intake this way, too.

The drawback for most diets is that one gets bored eating the same things over and over. Most people are tempted by the things that they can't eat and end up giving up on their diet altogether. Including all food groups stops this cycle of boredom and bingeing, and people find it easier to stick to a diet where you are allowed to have treats a few times a week.

Sodium is not bad, fats are not bad, and sugar is not bad, but when we overindulge in these things, they become bad for us.

Some tips to integrate the DASH diet into your everyday life include:

- Consider your portion size.

- Try and add as much color to your plate as possible.

- Every protein should have at least two different kinds of vegetable sides to accompany it.

- Be conscious about what is in your food.

- Opt for fruit for desserts and sweets treat rather than pastries and candy.

- Plan what you are going to eat in advance.

- Focus on your overall eating plan instead of just specific meals. This way, you will be able to get a variety of nutrients into your daily consumption.

Foods That Are Beneficial - Different Food Groups

Below is a graph showing how much of each food group to include in your daily diet:

The food groups were designed to differentiate between different types of foods. Foods that have similar reactions in the body and serve similar purposes will be grouped in the same category. Consuming specific amounts of each group is what keeps a person healthy since we need each of them to create a balanced diet.

The DASH diet also encourages people to eat more foods that are high in magnesium, calcium and potassium, as these are known to lower blood pressure.

Carbohydrates:

Carbs have gotten a bad reputation in the dieting world because people are under the false impression that they are what causes weight gain. Removing carbs completely from your diet is actually very unhealthy since carbohydrates are what are burned to create energy for your body to use.

However there are unhealthy carbs that can be avoided since they just create empty calories. These include highly processed breads and sugars.

Fat:

This is another food group that people tend to avoid because the name is something that people are trying to lose. But it is important to remember that there are good fats and bad fats. The bad fats are saturated fats and they have little to no nutritional value. These are the ones that stick in your body and create problems for your heart. Good fats actually increase overall health, and the body needs these in moderation.

Some examples of these include:

- Olive oil

- Avocados

- Nuts

- Hemp Seeds

- Flax seeds

- Fish rich in omega 3 fatty acids

Protein:

Yet again this is another food group that people tend to fixate on. Many diets recently have been developed around high protein. While protein is good for you, an excess of it is not. On the other hand, limiting it is not great for you either. You should be consuming a moderate amount of various proteins. Protein is what helps heal the body and build muscle.

Another misconception about protein is that you can only get good amounts of it in meat. The truth is that plants are a very good source of protein, and they are healthier because they have other nutrients in them. You also don't run the risk of the added preservatives that you find in many meats and processed meat products. If you do choose animal proteins, then it is good to make sure that they are not processed but are as pure and lean as possible.

Some healthy sources of proteins are:

- Legumes

- Soy products

- Nuts and seeds

- Lean meat

- Low-fat dairy

- Eggs

- Fish

Foods To Avoid

The DASH diet is very inclusive in that it does not state specifically to not eat any food group but rather includes all food groups in varying proportions. Obviously some food groups naturally have more nutrients and are more beneficial as a whole than others. Foods that do not fall in this category are the ones that need to be limited.

The DASH diet limits your intake of red meat, fat, sugar and salt. These foods are not completely cut out but rather enjoyed in a controlled manner so as not to have any negative effects on the body.

Processed foods are very high in sodium since it is used as a preservative to help food last longer on the shelf. The problem here is that the nutrients have been stripped away and overly processed junk is what is left. Most canned foods have little to no nutritional value, so you are just consuming empty calories. A good rule of thumb is, if you can't pronounce the ingredients on the label you shouldn't put it in your body. Natural ingredients will be written as what they are, but chemicals and preservatives always have long scientific names that you have probably never heard of before.

The point is not to cut out salt completely but rather to limit it to a healthy dosage per day. The body needs sodium to function, but too much of it can have multiple negative effects on the body. Make sure you don't cut it out completely, but rather keep it within the boundaries of healthy sodium intake.

Serving and Portion Sizes

Most people focus on what they are eating and neglect to consider how much of it they are eating. When talking about weight loss, it is important to note that you will not be able to lose any weight unless you are eating at a caloric deficit. What this means is that the calories you consume are less than the calories you are burning. If you are eating more than you are burning, you will gain weight, whether the calories are from a cheeseburger and chocolate milkshake or a mountain of kale salad.

In saying this, not all calories are created equal. Foods high in saturated fat contain a lot of calories per serving as opposed to nutrient-dense foods which usually carry fewer calories per serving. If you eat low-fat and high-nutrient foods, you will be able to eat more of it because the calories are lower. These foods will give you energy throughout the day and help you to feel fuller for longer.

The amount of food and calories one should consume varies from person to person. Age slows down your metabolism, so older people generally have to consume less than younger people.

Your level of activity should also be taken into consideration. Highly active people will have to eat more calories to sustain them, and people who lead a more sedentary life will need to consume less since less energy is being expended. Other factors to consider are weight, height and gender.

For example, a 60-year-old retired women could probably get away with eating about 1400-1600 calories a day. On the other hand, a 25-year-old man who plays sports as his leisure activity and is generally highly active will need about 2800-3000 calories to sustain him. If either of these two people wanted to lose weight, they would have to limit their calorie intake to about 500 calories less than they are burning. You can see how that would look different for each of them.

As an example of how calories can play a part in portion and serving sizes, the following table shows how someone who burns 1600 calories and someone who burns 2000 calories will need to alter their diets to fit their caloric needs. Bear in mind that this is the recommended serving for maintaining your current weight and not losing weight.

The serving sizes for each food will vary. If you are eating packaged food, then the recommended serving size will be on the package along with the caloric information.

Exercises To Aid Weight Loss

Exercise is vitally important in any weight-loss journey. It helps you to lose weight faster as well as toning your body and giving you more energy. As we exercise, we burn calories and work our muscles. If you are only trying to maintain your current weight, then you will be able to consume more calories when you have regular exercise in your routine.

For many people exercise is not something that they want to add into their routine. This can be because of busy schedules, being tired at the end of the day and just wanting to relax or simply it is just too hard. The truth is that there are many exercises that are not difficult or time-consuming that can have a huge positive effect on you.

The exercises in this chapter are easy to do and fit into most schedules. The truth is that most things that are good for us will require some effort and sacrifice and exercise is no different, so bear in mind that as simple as these are, they will require some effort. With that said, the benefits far outweigh the time and energy put in.

Walking

Walking is the perfect beginner's exercise. It is low-impact, and almost everyone is capable of doing it. It is also easy to integrate into your daily life. You are guaranteed to be walking for some portion of the day. The trick is to extend this time as much as you can.

Some tips to include walking in your daily routine are:

- Park farther away from your destination.

- Take the stairs instead of the elevator.

- Consciously take the long way to get somewhere instead of shorter ways.

- Set an alarm to take a walk around the building or outside every 1-2 hours.

- Take your dog or kids for a walk.

- Simply block out 20 minutes of your morning or evening to take a walk.

Jogging or Running

This is just a step above walking. If you feel like you are not ready to jump into jogging or running, you can start by walking and slowly increase the pace every week. A 20 to 30-minute run a few times a week has been shown to decrease belly fat in a few weeks.

Running lifts your heart rate and makes you sweat more, so you don't have to run lengthy amounts of time to reap the benefits. Block out 20-30 minutes 3-4 times a week or a morning or afternoon jog and your body will thank you.

Swimming

This is the perfect summer activity if you have a pool or are in close proximity to one. Swimming hardly ever feels like exercise since the water takes the pressure off your bones and muscles, however the resistance caused by the water helps you work your muscles and tone your body. Even just treading water for 30 minutes burns close to 400 calories.

Jumping Rope

Jumping rope for 20 minutes a few times a week has a significant impact on weight loss. It increases your heart rate and melts fat, and you don't even have to leave the living room. This exercise is perfect for those who don't want to leave the house. You can put on your favorite TV series and jump rope for those minutes. Jumping rope has similar benefits to running since they both spike your heart rate.

Chapter 11 Losing Weight with DASH Diet

Although the DASH diet was not formally created as a weight loss diet, it does promote weight loss. This is due to the DASH diets food groups and guidelines.

The well-balanced blend of nutritious low-calorie whole foods helps your body drop unnecessary weight.

There are three things about the DASH diet that make it particularly great for weight loss:

- Consuming healthy fats and omitting unhealthy fats

- High fiber intake

- High vitamin C intake

Choose low-calorie foods

You can lose weight on the DASH diet by eating foods that have fewer calories. The key to losing weight is to burn more calories than you eat in a day.

Exchange sweets and other high-calorie foods for low-calorie foods like fruits and vegetables. Eat smarter, eat smaller portions, eat slowly, and be a smart shopper.

Low-fat frozen yogurt will save you nearly 70 calories when compared to full-fat ice cream. Buy low-fat or fat-free when it is available and cut back on portion size.

If you want a snack, choose fresh fruit rather than a cookie or candy. This will increase your fruit consumption and save you about 80 calories per snack.

Dried fruits are a better choice than chips or pork rinds and will save you about 230 calories per snack.

If you have to buy canned fruit, make sure it is packaged in water and not syrup.

Plan ahead

Buy an assortment of vegetables, slice them, and take them to work along with a sandwich. This will increase your vegetable consumption, and it will help you resist the temptation to grab a bag of chips from the vending machine at lunch. Replacing a bag of chips with vegetables will save you about 120 calories.

Choose healthy snacks

Eat healthy snacks without adding unhealthy seasonings. Try popcorn cooked in olive oil and seasoned with garlic or grated parmesan cheese rather than butter and salt.

Choose water

Drink water with a twist of lemon or lime rather than sodas and sweetened teas.

Adhere to recommended serving sizes

Watch your serving sizes on labels.

Consume less sodium

Sodium will make you retain water, and it will cause inflammatory responses throughout your body. You need some sodium but not a lot.

Set a goal to watch your sodium intake and start paying attention to the information on food labels.

Prepackaged foods can contain excessive amounts of sodium.

Aim to buy foods that do not have salt added to them.

Watch the salt content in canned foods, sauces, tomato juices, and prepared foods.

Be creative and exchange salt with exotic spices when cooking meals. Let salt be your last resort.

The DASH diet provides guidelines for your sodium and caloric intake.

The standard DASH diet allows up to a maximum of 2300 mg of sodium per day, and the low-sodium version of the DASH diet allows up to 1500 mg of sodium per day.

The average American diet contains up to 3500 mg of sodium per day.

Go low-fat

Choose lower-fat methods of preparing your food such as baking, broiling, and grilling.

Also, reduce the amount of oil and margarine that you use when cooking and use low-fat condiments.

Be smart about eating out

Do some research on the restaurant that you are going to by looking them up online to see how they prepare their food. View their menu online as well.

Look for low sodium foods, low-fat, low calorie, and special areas on the menu that offer lighter meal plans. If you do not see them ask your server.

DASH Diet and Blood Pressure

This diet is centered along controlling salt intake as well as limiting the consumption of cholesterol and saturated fats, both of which are high contributors to heart diseases. It also focuses on increasing the taking of whole grains and fresh fruits, resulting in effective results while following this diet plan. It is highly recommended that those using it must combine it with other healthy lifestyle approaches like exercising, losing weight, reducing alcohol consumption, and possibly stop smoking altogether.

Dash Diet and Diabetes

Diabetes is mainly caused by insulin resistance. The DASH diet is tried and tested in curbing insulin resistance. If you're already suffering from diabetes, you can be certain of experiencing some relief. For those predisposed to the disease due to genetic factors, this can only prevent or delay the onset of diabetes.

Dash diet for Busy People

Trying to cram all your activities into a 24-hour day leaves very little time for food preparation. A busy lifestyle leads people to rely on fast food for their meals. Unfortunately, the most convenient solution for busy people can also be the unhealthiest option. Junk food has too much sodium, sugar and fat, and consuming it regularly can lead to many health issues like obesity and diabetes. The best approach to staying healthy even during hectic days is to plan ahead and acquire as much nutritional knowledge as possible.

Store nutritional snacks

Nuts and granola bars are far better options than chips and cookies. Carry healthy snacks to work and avoid relying on the vending machine for food. It's easy to be tempted to eat delicious but unhealthy food right after a busy workday. Having a stash of healthy snacks at home will lessen the urge to stop by the fast-food chain. You can use a Sunday to make a large batch of these healthy snacks. Just store them in containers and decide which one you'll consume each day.

Stick to your list

People benefit from mastering their grocery shopping. Try to list all the supplies needed for an entire week so that you'll spend less time on shopping. Try to stick to the list and avoid wandering off to the processed food section of the grocery store to avoid impulsive buying. You can also enlist the help of a friend or your partner when you go shopping. Not only will it take you less time to finish, but you'll also have help in staying away from the processed foods.

You must use the refrigerator

Cook meals that can be refrigerated. This way, you only have to cook once, and the dish can last for at least a few days. Set aside a few hours on Sunday nights to prepare meals for the week. Cook, divide into portions and refrigerate. This is the same thing as cutting your vegetables in bulk and placing them under cling film. Adding a little vinegar will help preserve your dishes longer, and you need not rely on salt to help your meals stay fresh.

Transform Your leftovers

Protein foods like chicken and pork can be reinvented in a number of ways. Although salads are the go-to dishes for leftovers, meat can be used in tortillas or sliced into small bits and added to low-sodium, low-fat mayonnaise for a sandwich. There are many different possibilities for leftovers; it is up to you to creatively transform one food into another to avoid getting bored eating the same dish over and over again. However, your leftovers will remain fresh only so long, and it is best to use today's leftovers only for the next couple of days.

Drink a lot of water

Busy people tend to forget to drink enough liquid, and oftentimes if they do drink, they choose soda or an energy drink. These contain too much sugar and can contribute to developing hypertension or diabetes. Also, watch out for calories inside commercially prepared drinks such as fruit juices, sweets or carbonated tea, and canned coffee. They also contain too much sugar and have a lot of empty calories, which can sabotage any diet plan. If your workplace does not have a water cooler for employees, bring a water bottle to work filled with water or plain tea. You can also choose fruit infused water, which serves the dual purpose of providing your body with the goodness of fresh fruits and water.

Keep Fit

When it comes to controlling your blood pressure, it is important to exercise regularly. This helps in reducing the amount of pressure that is exerted on the heart. Remember that your heart needs exercise, and you must engage in cardio to give it a thorough burn. Many people refrain from undertaking cardio exercise as they think it will tire them out completely. But the main aim of cardio is to exhaust you and help you achieve a burn. Apart from cardio, you must also do other forms of exercise, including lifting weights, core training, sides, back muscle stimulation, etc. After you do these, your body will be able to pump blood through your heart more easily.

Successful Tips for DASH Diet

Ease your way into a DASH diet lifestyle by using these helpful tips.

Change slowly

If you consume a given number of servings of a particular meal, e.g., vegetables and fruits, try to increase one more serving during lunch and/or dinner.

Make one or two of the grains you eat whole grains instead of changing all of them gradually.

Increasing whole grains, vegetables, and fruits slowly is important as it prevents the occurrence of diarrhea or bloating if you do not eat a diet high in fiber.

Be cautious with the food labels

You are heavily fighting sodium in this diet. When shopping, read labels. Here's the secret. If a label says "reduced sodium," run for your dear life. Reduced sodium does not mean its low. Low sodium diet has 140mg of sodium per serving. The recommended daily sodium intake per day is less than 2,300 mg.

Reward accomplishments and forgive mistakes

For the achievements you make, treat yourself to rewards that are nonfood. These include buying a book, spending time with a friend, or renting a movie.

The human being is to error. You will also, one time or another, make mistakes. Accept that and avoid it happening again.

Cook at home

Eating out does not give you many healthy options. You may scrutinize the menu to the very last option, but you can't really tell the ingredients in every meal. A vegetarian option may be the closest you'll get to a meal that adheres to the DASH diet.

Why not prepare your own meals at home? No matter how busy you are, you sure can squeeze in an extra hour that will have a positive impact on your health. Start by looking for interesting recipes then shopping for the ingredients. That will get you in the mood for cooking. Cook a lot of food at a time and refrigerate/freeze in portions, so you do not have to cook from scratch each time. Chop the vegetables before refrigerating them, so you can have them ready in minutes when you need them.

Make exercise an important part of your DASH diet lifestyle

The DASH diet eating plan will improve your health and make you lose weight all on its own. However, if you make regular exercise a habit, you will boost your body's ability to shed unwanted pounds.

When you combine DASH diet eating with a good amount of physical activity (30 minutes/day of moderate exercise), it will also maximize your ability to reduce blood pressure.

Get Company

Join a community of other people following the DASH diet. Here you will trade experiences, share recipes, gauge progress, and generally get adequate support.

For all the benefits it harbors, the DASH diet is well worth the effort. With time, you even forget that you're on a diet, you simply turn healthy eating into a lifestyle. And for that, you increase your chances of lifelong wellness of body and mind.

Frequently Asked Questions About DASH Diet

Is the DASH diet for only people with hypertension?

No. although it was designed for people with hypertension, the diet has been adopted by several other groups for its benefits in ameliorating their health conditions. This includes people who are trying to lose weight, build lean muscle, etc. Along with a substantial reduction in weight, DASH dieters also see their hypertension reduced, which helps them lead happy lives free from stress and illness.

Does the diet follow a phase system?

Yes. It follows a two-phase system where the first phase completely eliminates foods that are starchy and laden with carbohydrates, and the second phase slowly reintroduces them. This system helps the person's body cope with the diet so they can continue with it for a long time. The two phases have a difference of 2 weeks between them, and that is the time when dieters are said to experience the greatest amount of weight loss.

Does DASH diet help to lose weight?

Yes. This diet is said to be quite effective in helping people lose weight. It is said to be on par with some of the other diets that are prescribed specifically for weight loss, and if followed the right way, it can have the same results on people's bodies. The diet is quite effective not just in helping a person lose weight but also in keeping that weight from coming back. The diet can be seen as your one-stop, ultra-effective means to cut down on excess weight and maintain a healthy body.

Is it ideal for children and adults?

The diet can be followed by people above the age of 18. Children below that age might need foods rich in carbs and salt for proper growth. Anybody else looking to reduce their high blood pressure and hypertension and cut down on their weight can take up the diet. There is no upper age limit for the diet. However, older people need to check with their doctors first to know if it will be safe for them to take up the diet.

Are the results fast?

The results will depend on how seriously you take the diet – whether you are strictly following the rules of the diet and are incorporating only the allowed food items. The results can usually be seen within the first month of the diet, but it will vary from person to person. It can be fast for some and might take some more time for others. If you are taking up the diet with another person, then it is best that you not compare your results with theirs and focus only on your diet.

Can the results be noticed?

Yes. The results are quite easy to see, and you will feel that your blood pressure has dropped and your metabolism is now much better. You will feel a physical change and feel lighter after taking up the diet. The diet will also help you maintain a slim figure and give you a chance to build lean, strong muscles. You will see a reduction in your waistline, and this will help bring down your blood pressure. You will feel much more energetic and capable of doing physical tasks without exerting too much pressure on your heart.

Can vegetarians enjoy the perks of a DASH diet?

It is flexible for various food preferences. Vegetarians can also enjoy the benefits of a DASH diet while keeping up their meat and dairy products aversions. In the DASH diet, there is a number of vegetarian options available, which mainly includes grains, fruits, beans, and veggies.

Conclusion

Dash Diet has gained popularity in the past few years as it is extremely helpful in strengthening metabolism and controlling hypertension. Contrary to the popular belief that while following the dash diet, one gets to only eat vegetarian foods while you get a balanced diet that includes fresh fruits, vegetables, nuts, low-fat dairy products and whole grains. You do not have to completely cut down on meat instead you just have to reduce sodium and fat content from your everyday diet.

The diet also has many health benefits as it helps in reducing hypertension and obesity lowering osteoporosis and preventing cancer. This well-balanced diet strengthens metabolism which further helps in decomposing the fat deposits stored in the body. This, in turn, improves the overall health of a person.

This book provides a 21-day meal plan with snack options for midmornings and midafternoons. However, you can consult experts in case you suffer from contemporary health conditions or follow certain exercise routines; as this will help you customize the diet as per your requirement.

This diet is easy to follow as you get to everything but in a healthier fashion and limited quantity.

Talking about the DASH diet outside the theory and more in practice reveals more of its efficiency as a diet. Besides excess research and experiments, the true reasons of people looking into this diet are its certain features. It gives the feeling of ease and convenience, which makes the users more comfortable with its rules and regulations.

Here some of the reasons why the DASH Diet works amazingly:

1. Easy to Adopt:

The broad range of options available under the label of DASH diet makes it more flexible for all. This is the reason that people find it easier to switch to and harness its true health benefits. It makes adaptability easier for its users.

2. Promotes Exercise:

It is most effective than all the other factors because not only does it focus on the food and its intake, but it also duly stresses daily exercises and routine physical activities. This is the reason that it produces quick, visible results.

3. All Inclusive:

With few limitations, this Diet has taken every food item into its fold with certain modifications. It rightly guides about the Dos and Don'ts of all the ingredients and prevents us from consuming those which are harmful to the body and its health.

4. A Well Balanced Approach:

One of its biggest advantages is that it maintains balance in our diet, in our routine, our caloric intake, and our nutrition.

5. Good Caloric Check:

Every meal we plan on the DASH diet is pre-calculated in terms of calories. We can easily keep track of the daily caloric intake and consequently restrict them easily by cutting off certain food items.

6. Prohibits Bad Food:

The DASH diet suggests the use of more organic and fresh food and discourages the use of processed food and junk items available in stores. So, it creates better eating habits in the users.

7. Focused on Prevention:

Though it is proven to be a cure for many diseases, it is described as more of a preventive strategy.

8. Slow Yet Progressive Changes:

The diet is not highly restrictive and accommodates gradual changes towards achieving the ultimate health goal. You can set up your daily, weekly, or even monthly targets at your own convenience.

9. Long Term Effects:

The results of the DASH diet are not just incredible, but they are also long-lasting. It is considered slow in progress, but the effects last longer.

10. Accelerates Metabolism:

With its healthy approach to life, the DASH diet has the ability to activate our metabolism and boost it for better functioning of the body.

DASH DIET COOKBOOK FOR BEGINNERS:

140 OF THE GREATEST DASH DIET RECIPES DESIGNED TO MAKE YOU LOSE WEIGHT AND LOWER YOUR BLOOD PRESSURE. UNCONVENTIONAL DISHES TO START ENJOYING HEALTHY FOOD.

BEATRICE MORELLI

Introduction

Thank you for choosing this diet book, I hope you are ready to make the delicious dash diet recipes. I have also prepared another book in which the DASH diet is widely discussed, *DASH Diet for Beginners: Learn How the 21-Day DASH Diet Meal Plan Is Proven to Make You Lose Weight and Lower Your Blood Pressure. Improve Your Health and Live a Better Life.*

The DASH diet leans heavily on vegetables, fruits, and whole grains. Fish and lean poultry are served moderately. Whole wheat flour is used instead of white flour. Using salt is discouraged. Instead, participants are encouraged to season foods with spices and herbs to add flavor without adding salt. DASH as a diet plan promotes the consumption of low-fat dairy, lean meat, fruits, and vegetables. It is literally a mix of old world and new world eating plans. It has been designed to follow old world diet principles to help eliminate new world health problems.

The carbohydrates are mainly made of plant fiber which the body does not easily digest and therefore cannot turn into stored fat. The plan is rich in good fats that make food taste good and help us feel fuller for a longer period of time. Proteins are not forbidden but are geared more toward plant-based protein and not so much meat consumption.

When filling the plate for a meal, it is important that the food be attractive as well as tasty and nutritious. A wide variety of foods will make this plan much more interesting. Try to make choices that will offer a range of colors and textures. And remember that dessert is not off limits but should be based around healthy choices that include fresh fruit.

The DASH eating plans emphasis on vegetables, fruits, whole grains, and low-fat dairy products makes it an ideal plan for anyone looking to gain health through lowered blood pressure and a healthier heart. It is a heart healthy way of eating. The DASH plan has no specialized recipes or food plans. Daily caloric intake depends on a person's activity level and age. People who need to lose weight would naturally eat fewer calories.

The DASH diet's major focus is on grains, vegetables, and fruits because these foods are higher fiber foods and will make you feel full longer. Whole grains should be consumed six to eight times daily, vegetables four to six servings daily, and fruit four to five servings daily. Low-fat dairy is an important part of the diet and should be eaten two to three times daily. And there should be six or fewer servings daily of fish, poultry, and lean meat. The DASH diet does not limit red meat the way the Mediterranean diet does, but it still keeps it lean.

Chapter 1 Health Benefits And Why It Works

How DASH Diet works

The food plan mainly focuses on vegetables, fruits, low-fat/non-Fat dairy, and whole grains. The eating plan also includes the consumption of high fiber foods, medium to low amounts of fat, low red meat, and less sugar. An additional benefit of this diet is that it is rich in different vitamins and minerals that are important in achieving a healthy body.

Another good thing about this diet plan is that it lowers your Sodium intake in your diet (daily consumption for Sodium is only 2,3oo mg on the dash diet) that will help regulate blood pressure levels. That's because studies show that eating food with high sodium content could lead to a spike in blood pressure.

The diet plan has claimed to lower the blood pressure in just two weeks and has been recommended by Centers for Disease Control, American Heart Association, The National Heart, Lungand Blood Institute, the Mayo Clinic, US Government guidelines for the treatment of hypertension and a lot more.

History of DASH Diet

DASH diet dates back to the early 1990s when concern was raised about the prevalence of lifestyle diseases, among them hypertension. In 1992, under the funding of the National Institute of Health (NIH), several research projects were initiated to determine if dietary changes could be effective in treating hypertension.

The participants were provided with a meal plan and advised not to include any other lifestyle modification so that all the changes could be attributed directly to the dietary interventions.

The results were encouraging. A decrease of about 6 to 11 mm Hg was reported in systolic blood pressure in a span of a few weeks. In addition, the lower levels of Sodium in the diet dropped, the lower the blood pressure dropped. In addition to reducing hypertension, the cholesterol levels were reduced as well.

After several subsequent studies and experiments with positive results, the DASH diet became and still is highly recommended as a long-term remedy for hypertension.

The DASH Diet is touted for its many health benefits. Perhaps one of the most important benefits of this particular diet is that it can help stabilize the blood pressure levels of hypertensive people. Because this particular diet is low in

Sodium, it can help go down the systolic blood pressure levels by up to 14 points. But more than benefit hypertensive individuals, the DASH Diet also comes with many advantages.

The DASH diet comes with a range of health benefits. Following are some of the major advantages of following the DASH diet: Cardiovascular Health

The DASH diet decreases your consumption of refined carbohydrates by increasing your consumption of foods high in potassium and dietary fiber (fruits, vegetables, and whole grains). In addition, it diminishes your consumption of saturated fats. Therefore, the DASH diet has a favorable effect on your lipid profile and glucose tolerance, which reduces the prevalence of metabolic syndrome (MS) in post-menopausal women.

Reports state that a diet limited to 500 calories favors a loss of 17% of total body weight in 6 months in overweight women. This reduces the prevalence of MS by 15%. However, when this diet follows the patterns of the DASH diet, while triglycerides decrease in a similar way, the reduction in weight and BP is even greater.

It also reduces blood sugar and increases HDL, which decreases the prevalence of MS in 35% of women. These results contrast with those of other studies, which have reported that the DASH diet alone, i.e., without caloric restriction, does not affect HDL and glycemia. This means that the effects of the DASH diet on MS are associated mainly with the greater reduction in BP and that, for more changes, the diet would be required to be combined with weight loss.

Helpful for Patients with Diabetes

The DASH diet has also been shown to help reduce inflammatory and coagulation factors (C-reactive protein and fibrinogen) in patients with diabetes. These benefits are associated with the contribution of antioxidants and fibers, given the high consumption of fruits and vegetables that the DASH diet requires. In addition, the DASH diet has been shown to reduce total cholesterol and LDL, which reduces the estimated 10-year cardiovascular risk. Epidemiological studies have determined that women in the highest quintile of food consumption according to the DASH diet have a 24% to 33% lower risk of coronary events and an 18% lower risk of a cerebrovascular event. Similarly, a meta-analysis of six observational studies has determined that the DASH diet can reduce the risk of cardiovascular events by 20%.

Weight Reduction

Limited research associates the DASH diet, in isolation, with weight reduction. In some studies, weight reduction was greater when the subject was on the DASH diet as compared to an isocaloric controlled diet. This could be related to the higher calcium intake and lower energy density of the DASH diet. The American guidelines for the treatment of obesity emphasize that, regardless of diet, a caloric restriction would be the most important factor in reducing weight.

However, several studies have made an association between 1. greater weight and fat loss in diets and 2. caloric restriction and higher calcium intake. Studies have also observed an inverse association between dairy consumption and body mass index (BMI). In obese patients, weight loss has been reported as being 170% higher after 24 weeks on a hypocaloric diet with high calcium intake.

In addition, the loss of trunk fat was reported to be 34% of the total weight loss as compared to only 21% in a control diet. It has also been determined that a calcium intake of 20 mg per gram has a protective effect in overweight middle-aged women. This would be equivalent to 1275 mg of calcium for a western diet of 1700 kcal. It has been suggested that low calcium intake increases the circulating level of the parathyroid hormone and vitamin D, which have been shown to increase the level of cytosolic calcium in adipocytes in vitro, changing the metabolism of lipolysis to lipogenesis. Despite these reports, the effect that diet-provided calcium has on women's weight after menopause is a controversial subject. An epidemiological study has noted that a sedentary lifestyle and, to a lesser extent, caloric intake are associated with post-menopausal weight gain, though calcium intake is not associated with it. The average calcium intake in this group of women is approximately 1000 mg which would be low, as previously stated. Another study of post-menopausal women shows that calcium and vitamin D supplementation in those with a calcium intake of less than 1200 mg per day decreases the risk of weight gain by 11%.

 In short, the DASH diet is favorable, both in weight control and in the regulation of fatty tissue deposits, due to its high calcium content (1200 mg/day). The contribution of calcium apparently plays a vital role in the regulation of lipogenesis.

• Increased intake of important micronutrients: While this particular diet discourages the intake of

Sodium, it promotes the consumption of foods that are rich in Magnesium, Calcium, and Potassium. Thus, those who follow this particular diet regimen can increase their intake of important micronutrients, thereby preventing nutrient deficiency.

• May promote weight loss: Aside from reducing the intake of sodium, the DASH Diet may promote weight loss because it encourages people to eat foods that are rich in fiber and low in calories such as fruits, vegetables, and whole grains. This diet also limits the consumption of too much protein and fats; thus, it can help people who want to lose weight.

• Stabilize blood glucose levels: The DASH Diet encourages people to consume good carbs in the form of complex carbohydrates that are rich in fiber. Complex carbohydrates take time to be converted into glucose. This also allows the body to be able to utilize the glucose to feed the cells and fewer opportunities for it to be converted into glucagon in the liver and muscles.

• Healthier kidneys: It is crucial to take note that high blood pressure is related to kidney diseases. The reduced intake of salt can help reduce the likelihood of kidney stone formation. This particular diet is supported by the National Kidney Foundation.

• Better bone health: This particular diet encourages the consumption of Calcium; thus, it can help improve bone health. This diet will benefit people who may suffer from osteoporosis.

• Better heart health and cholesterol level: The DASH Diet is somewhat restrictive to the kind of fats that you take in. In fact, you are only allowed to use small amounts of oil for this particular diet but are encouraged to take in good fats such as olive oil and Omega-3 fatty acids for better heart health and good cholesterol level in the body.

Chapter 2 Dash Diet Tips

Tips For Healthy Eating On The Run

Absence of time is a significant motivation behind why numerous individuals forego healthy eating. Inexpensive food is promptly accessible and it's temptingly modest and filling. While eating inexpensive food is never as healthy as a well-arranged, adjusted diet, if you should eat cheap food, you can without much of a stretch find a way to improve the nature of your nourishment when on the run.

Watch divide sizes. Your hankering will probably be fulfilled after you have completed a little request of fries, and you'll spare more than 100 calories when contrasted and the supersized request. Similar remains constant for sandwiches. Request the normal form or even a child's dinner for yourself.

Search out store style inexpensive food chains where you can arrange a sub or sandwich on entire wheat bread or a wrap, a lower fat and lower-calorie alternative than singed food.

Some cheap food chains currently offer healthy sides instead of the universal French fries. Take the healthy alternative. Or then again if you can't stand to surrender the oil and salt, get the healthy side request, as well.

Continuously request a side serving of mixed greens when eating at customary inexpensive food outlets. You will be less inclined to top off on just the unhealthy things, and the serving of mixed greens will give some fiber and nutrients to adjust a generally unhealthy supper.

Recollect that chicken isn't constantly a healthy decision. Some cheap food chains offer seared breaded chicken sandwiches on white bread that are really more extravagant in fat and calories than a burger. Flame broiled chicken is a superior choice.

Make it a propensity to eat a bit of natural product, a bowl of oat, or some low fat yogurt before you set out to get things done. Customary eating can assist you with feeling full and keep away from allurement.

Stock your vehicle with filtered water and healthy bites. Have a little nibble before the yearnings hit and you're more averse to maneuver into that drive-through inexpensive food outlet.

Consider a store for your cheap food break. You can get precut and washed crisp natural product or vegetables, yogurt, or low fat cheddar. Numerous general stores additionally offer sushi, wraps, plates of mixed greens, or other healthy arranged things.

Hold the mayo. A tablespoon of standard mayonnaise has just about 100 calories!

Try not to include a sugary, calorie-rich beverage to an effectively unhealthy feast. Water is accessible all over the place and is beneficial for you. Drinking a huge glass of water with your dinner will assist you with feeling more full prior.

Probably the greatest obstruction to healthy eating is an absence of time, which is the thing that demoralizes numerous individuals from making the jump to eat significantly more healthily. Because cheap food and shoddy nourishment has all the earmarks of being significantly more promptly accessible than healthy choices, numerous individuals just surrender to the allurement and eat ineffectively during their bustling days.

What numerous individuals don't understand is that it just takes a smidgen of pre-wanting to guarantee that suppers and tidbits are healthy during the day. Coming up next are a few hints which will assist you with deciding on the healthier eating decisions during your occupied, distressing day.

1. Ensure you eat your foods grown from the ground for the afternoon.

The best part about foods grown from the ground is that a large number of them are incredibly versatile. Keep a few bits of natural product, or some cut vegetables in your vehicle or on your office work area. When you are feeling hungry, pick these healthy snacks as opposed to making the trek to the candy machine or halting at a comfort store for a sugary tidbit.

2. Regardless of where you eat, ensure that you are watching your bit sizes.

You ought to consistently settle on the littler, if not the littlest, size for your supper. If you completely should have those salty French fries, decide on the littlest size because it will more than likely be sufficient to control your hankering without going too over the edge as far as calories.

3. If you are on the run and have no different alternatives however inexpensive food...

.Attempt to discover a shop style area as opposed to halting at the nearest drive-through. Submarine sandwiches on entire wheat or wraps are alternatives which are a lot of lower both in calories and fat than what you would have found at another cheap food area.

4. Most places offer healthy sides which you should exploit.

There are numerous different alternatives accessible to you that are just much preferable for you over French fries. Numerous spots considerably offer servings of mixed greens now, which while not as healthy as a plate of mixed greens you would make at home, can undoubtedly check your appetite without overpowering you with such a large number of calories.

5. Pick flame broiled alternatives whenever they are accessible.

Chicken might be a healthy decision as a rule, yet the seared and breaded chicken decisions that many drive-through joints offer are in reality high in calories and fat. Settle on a flame broiled chicken sandwich.

6. Stop at a grocery store on your mid-day break, rather than a drive-through eatery.

Supermarkets offer many brisk food alternatives, similar to vegetables and natural product which are as of now washed and cut and separately bundled, or little submarine sandwiches with the toppings as an afterthought. If you snatch a sandwich, make sure to get a yogurt cup or an individual bit of natural product too for a balanced noon feast.

7. Discussing sauces, attempt to maintain a strategic distance from mayonnaise if you can.

You may not understand this: A simple tablespoon of mayonnaise can have upwards of 100 calories! Yuck!

8. Keep water with you consistently.

Maintain a strategic distance from sugary beverages and beverages with a great deal of caffeine, rather settling on the healthiest thing that you can place into your body: Water. Keep filtered water in your vehicle, or a gallon container of water at the workplace with you. Water will likewise assist you with feeling full quicker, if you drink a huge glass before each bite or dinner.

Chapter 3 Best Diet Tips To Lose Weight And Improve Health

L et's be honest — there's a mind-boggling measure of data on the Internet about how to immediately shed pounds and get fit as a fiddle.

If you're searching for the best tips on the most proficient method to get in shape and keep it off, this apparently interminable measure of counsel can be overpowering and confounding.

From the diets elevating crude foods to dinner designs that rotate around shakes and prepackaged foods, another prevailing fashion diet appears to spring up each day.

The issue is, albeit prohibitive diets and disposal feast plans will in all likelihood bring about transient weight loss, the vast majority can't keep up them and wind up quitting inside half a month.

Despite the fact that shedding 10 pounds (4.5 kg) in seven days by following a prevailing fashion diet may appear to be enticing actually this sort of weight loss is often unhealthy and unsustainable.

The genuine key to sheltered and effective weight loss is to embrace a healthy lifestyle that suits your individual needs and that you can keep up forever.

The accompanying tips are healthy, practical approaches to get you in the groove again and headed towards your weight and wellness objectives.

Here are 25 of the best dieting tips to improve your health and assist you with getting more fit.

1. Top off on Fiber

Fiber is found in healthy foods including vegetables, organic products, beans and entire grains.

A few investigations have demonstrated that basically eating more fiber-rich foods may assist you with getting in shape and keep it off.

2. Jettison Added Sugar

Included sugar, particularly from sugary beverages, is a significant purpose behind unhealthy weight addition and health issues like diabetes and coronary illness.

Also, foods like treats, pop and prepared merchandise that contain heaps of added sugars will in general be low in the supplements your body needs to remain healthy.

Removing foods high in included sugars is an incredible method to lose overabundance weight.

It's imperative to take note of that even foods advanced as "healthy" or "natural" can be extremely high in sugar. Therefore, perusing nourishment marks is an absolute necessity.

3. Prepare for Healthy Fat

While fat is often the primary thing that gets slice when you're attempting to thin down, healthy fats can really assist you with arriving at your weight loss objectives.

Likewise, fats assist you with remaining more full for more, diminishing desires and helping you remain on track.

4. Limit Distractions

While expending dinners before your TV or PC may not appear as though diet harm, eating while diverted may make you devour more calories and put on weight.

Having during supper, away from potential interruptions, isn't just a decent method to hold your weight down — it likewise permits you an opportunity to reconnect with friends and family.

Cell phones are another gadget you should save while you're eating. Looking through messages or your Instagram or Facebook channel is similarly as diverting as a TV or PC.

5. Walk Your Way to Health

Numerous individuals accept they should receive a thorough exercise routine to kick off weight loss.

While different kinds of movement are significant when you're endeavoring to get fit as a fiddle, strolling is an astounding and simple approach to consume calories.

Actually, only 30 minutes of strolling every day has been appeared to help in weight loss.

Furthermore, it's an agreeable action that you can do both inside and outside whenever of day.

6. Draw out Your Inner Chef

Preparing more suppers at home has been appeared to advance weight loss and healthy eating.

Despite the fact that eating suppers at cafés is pleasant and can fit into a healthy diet plan, concentrating on preparing more dinners at home is an incredible method to hold your weight under tight restraints.

Furthermore, getting ready suppers at home enables you to explore different avenues regarding new, healthy fixings while setting aside you cash simultaneously.

7. Have a Protein-Rich Breakfast

Counting protein-rich foods like eggs in your morning meal has been appeared to profit weight loss.

Essentially swapping your everyday bowl of oat for a protein-pressed scramble made with eggs and sauteed veggies can assist you with shedding pounds.

Expanding protein consumption toward the beginning of the day may likewise assist you with staying away from unhealthy eating and improve hunger control for the duration of the day.

8. Try not to Drink Your Calories

While a great many people realize they ought to keep away from soft drinks and milkshakes, numerous individuals don't understand that even beverages publicized to support athletic execution or improve health can be stacked with undesirable fixings.

Sports drinks, espresso refreshments and enhanced waters will in general be extremely high in calories, artificial colorings and included sugar.

Indeed, even squeeze, which is often advanced as a healthy refreshment, can prompt weight gain if you devour excessively.

Concentrate on hydrating with water to limit the quantity of calories you drink for the duration of the day.

9. Shop Smart

Making a shopping rundown and adhering to it is an incredible method to abstain from purchasing unhealthy foods imprudently.

Also, making a shopping list has been appeared to prompt healthier eating and advance weight loss.

Another approach to restrict unhealthy buys at the market is to have a healthy supper or nibble before you go out to shop.

Studies have indicated that eager customers will in general reach for fattier, unhealthy foods.

10. Remain Hydrated

Drinking enough water for the duration of the day is useful for generally speaking health and can even assist you with keeping up a healthy weight.

One investigation of more than 9,500 individuals found that the individuals who were not enough hydrated had higher weight records (BMIs) and were bound to be hefty than the individuals who were appropriately hydrated (16).

Furthermore, individuals who drink water before suppers have been appeared to eat less calories.

11. Practice Mindful Eating

Hurrying through suppers or eating in a hurry may lead you to expend excessively, too rapidly.

Rather, be aware of your food, concentrating on how each nibble tastes. It might lead you to be increasingly mindful of when you are full, diminishing your odds of gorging (18).

Concentrating on eating gradually and making the most of your dinner, regardless of whether you have restricted time, is an extraordinary method to diminish gorging.

12. Cut Back on Refined Carbs

Refined carbs incorporate sugars and grains that have had their fiber and different supplements expelled. Models incorporate white flour, pasta and bread.

These sorts of foods are low in fiber, are processed rapidly and just keep you full for a brief timeframe.

Rather, pick wellsprings of complex sugars like oats, antiquated grains like quinoa and grain, or veggies like carrots and potatoes.

They'll help keep you more full for more and contain a lot a greater number of supplements than refined wellsprings of starches.

13. Lift Heavier to Get Lighter

Albeit high-impact practice like energetic strolling running and biking is fantastic for weight loss, numerous individuals will in general spotlight exclusively on cardio and don't add quality preparing to their schedules.

Adding weight lifting to your exercise center routine can assist you with building more muscle and tone your whole body.

Likewise, thinks about have indicated that weight lifting gives your digestion a little lift, helping you consume more calories for the duration of the day, in any event, when you are very still (20).

14. Set Meaningful Goals

Fitting into pants from secondary school or glancing better in a bathing suit are famous reasons why individuals need to get thinner.

Nonetheless, it's significantly more important to genuinely comprehend why you need to get in shape and the manners in which that weight loss may decidedly influence your life. Having these objectives as a top priority may assist you with adhering to your arrangement.

Having the option to play tag with your kids or having the stamina to move throughout the night at a friend or family member's wedding are instances of objectives that can keep you focused on a positive change.

15. Maintain a strategic distance from Fad Diets

Prevailing fashion diets are elevated for their capacity to assist individuals with shedding pounds quick.

Nonetheless, these diets will in general be extremely prohibitive and difficult to keep up. This prompts yo-yo dieting where individuals lose pounds, just to restore them.

While this cycle is basic in those attempting to take care of business rapidly, yo-yo dieting has been connected to a more noteworthy increment in body weight after some time.

Moreover, contemplates have demonstrated that yo-yo dieting can build the danger of diabetes, coronary illness, hypertension and metabolic disorder.

These diets might be enticing however finding a practical, healthy eating plan that sustains your body as opposed to denying it is a vastly improved decision.

16. Eat Whole Foods

Monitoring precisely what is going into your body is an extraordinary method to get healthy.

Eating entire foods that don't accompany a fixing list guarantees that you are supporting your body with normal, supplement thick foods.

When buying foods with fixing records, toning it down would be ideal.

If an item has heaps of fixings that you are new to, odds are it isn't the healthiest choice.

17. Pal Up

If you are experiencing difficulty adhering to an exercise normal or healthy eating plan, welcome a companion to go along with you and assist you with remaining on track.

Studies show that individuals who thin down with a companion are bound to stay with weight loss and exercise programs. They additionally will in general lose more weight than the individuals who go only it.

In addition, having a companion or relative with a similar health and wellbeing objectives can assist you with remaining spurred while having a fabulous time simultaneously.

18. Try not to Deprive Yourself

Disclosing to yourself that you will never have your preferred foods again isn't just ridiculous, however it might likewise set you up for disappointment.

Denying yourself will just make you need the prohibited food more and may make you gorge when you at long last collapse.

Accounting for suitable extravagances to a great extent will show you poise and prevent you from feeling angry of your new, healthy lifestyle.

Having the option to appreciate a little segment of a custom made sweet or enjoying a most loved occasion dish is a piece of having a healthy association with food.

19. Be Realistic

Contrasting yourself with models in magazines or famous people on TV isn't just unreasonable — it can likewise be unhealthy.

While having a healthy good example can be an extraordinary method to remain propelled, being excessively condemning of yourself can interfere with you and may prompt unhealthy practices.

Give centering a shot how you feel as opposed to focusing on what you look like. Your fundamental inspirations ought to be to get more joyful, fitter and healthier.

20. Veg Out

Vegetables are stacked with fiber and the supplements your body hungers for.

In addition, expanding your vegetable admission can assist you with getting more fit.

Truth be told, ponders show that just eating a serving of mixed greens before a supper can assist you with feeling full, making you eat less.

Moreover, topping off on veggies for the duration of the day can assist you with keeping up a healthy weight and may diminish your danger of creating interminable sicknesses like coronary illness and diabetes

21. Bite Smart

Nibbling on unhealthy foods can cause weight gain.

A simple method to help shed pounds or keep up a healthy weight is to attempt to have healthy snacks accessible at home, in your vehicle and at your work environment.

For instance, reserving pre-distributed servings of blended nuts in your vehicle or having cut-up veggies and hummus prepared in your refrigerator can assist you with remaining on track when a hankering strikes.

22. Fill the Void

Fatigue may lead you to go after unhealthy foods.

Studies have indicated that being exhausted adds to an expansion in generally calorie utilization because it impacts individuals to eat more food, healthy and unhealthy.

Finding new exercises or side interests that you appreciate is a great method to abstain from gorging brought about by weariness.

Essentially taking a walk and getting a charge out of nature can help show signs of improvement attitude to remain persuaded and adhere to your health objectives.

23. Set aside a few minutes for Yourself

Making a healthier lifestyle implies finding an opportunity to put yourself first, regardless of whether you don't believe it's conceivable.

Life often hinders weight loss and wellness objectives, so it is imperative to make an arrangement that incorporates individual time, and stick to it.

Obligations like work and child rearing are the absolute most significant things in life, however your health ought to be one of your top needs.

Regardless of whether that implies setting up a healthy lunch to bring to work, going for a run or going to a wellness class, putting aside time to deal with yourself can do ponders for both your physical and emotional wellness.

24. Discover Workouts You Actually Enjoy

The extraordinary thing about picking an exercise routine is that there are unlimited conceivable outcomes.

While perspiring through a turn class probably won't be some tea, mountain biking in a recreation center may be more suited to your abilities.

Certain exercises consume a larger number of calories than others. Be that as it may, you shouldn't pick an exercise dependent on the outcomes you think you'll get from it.

It's imperative to discover exercises that you anticipate doing and that satisfy you. That way you are bound to stay with them.

25. Backing Is Everything

Having a gathering of companions or relatives that supports you in your weight and wellbeing objectives is basic for effective weight loss.

Encircle yourself with constructive individuals who make you like making a healthy lifestyle will assist you with remaining spurred and on track.

Actually, thinks about have demonstrated that going to help gatherings and having a solid informal community assists individuals with getting in shape and keep it off (32).

Imparting your objectives to reliable and empowering loved ones can assist you with remaining responsible and set you up for progress.

If you don't have a strong family or gathering of companions, have a go at joining a care group. There are countless gatherings that meet face to face or on the web.

While there are numerous approaches to get in shape, finding a healthy eating and exercise plan that you can pursue for life is the most ideal approach to guarantee effective, long haul weight loss. In spite of the fact that prevailing fashion diets may offer a convenient solution, they are often unhealthy and deny the body of the supplements and calories it needs, driving the vast majority to come back to unhealthy propensities after they hit their weight loss objective.

Being progressively dynamic, concentrating on entire foods, decreasing included sugar and setting aside a few minutes for yourself are only a couple of approaches to get healthier and more joyful.

Keep in mind, weight loss isn't one-size-fits-all. To be fruitful, it is essential to discover an arrangement that works for you and fits well with your lifestyle.

It is anything but a win or bust procedure, either. If you can't focus on every one of the recommendations in this book, take a stab at beginning with only a not many that you think will work for you. They'll assist you with arriving at your health and wellbeing objectives in a protected and reasonable manner.

Chapter 4 Breakfast Recipes

Sweet Potatoes with Coconut Flakes

Preparation time: 15 mins

Cooking time: 1 hour

Servings: 2

Ingredients:

16 oz. sweet potatoes

1 tbsp. maple syrup

¼ c.

Fat-free coconut Greek yogurt

1/8 c. unsweetened toasted coconut flakes

1 chopped apple

Directions:

Preheat oven to 400 0F.

Place your potatoes on a baking sheet. Bake them for 45 - 60 minutes or until soft.

Use a sharp knife to mark "X" on the potatoes and fluff pulp with a fork.

Top with coconut flakes, chopped apple, Greek yogurt, and maple syrup.

Serve immediately.

Nutrition:

Calories: 321, Fat: 3 g Carbs: 70 g

Protein: 7 g Sugars: 0.1 g Sodium: 3%

Flaxseed & Banana Smoothie

Preparation time: 5 mins

Cooking time: 0 mins

Servings: 1

Ingredients:

1 frozen banana ½ c. almond milk

Vanilla extract. 1 tbsp. almond butter

2 tbsps. Flax seed 1 tsp. maple syrup

Directions:

Add all your ingredients to a food processor or blender and run until smooth. Pour the mixture into a glass and enjoy.

Nutrition:

Calories: 376, Fat:19.4 g Carbs:48.3 g

Protein:9.2 g Sugars:12% Sodium:64.9 mg

Fruity Tofu Smoothie

Preparation time: 5 mins

Cooking time: 0 mins

Servings: 2

Ingredients:

1 c. ice cold water

1 c. packed spinach

¼ c. frozen mango chunks

½ c. frozen pineapple chunks

1 tbsp. chia seeds

1 container silken tofu

1 frozen medium banana

Directions:

In a powerful blender, add all ingredients and puree until smooth and creamy.

Evenly divide into two glasses, serve and enjoy.

Nutrition: Calories: 175, Fat:3.7 g

Carbs:33.3 g Protein:6.0 g

Sugars:16.3 g Sodium:1%

French Toast with Applesauce

Preparation time: 5 mins

Cooking time: 5 mins

Servings: 6

Ingredients:

¼ c. unsweetened applesauce

½ c. skim milk

2 packets Stevia

2 eggs

6 slices whole wheat bread

1 tsp. ground cinnamon

Directions:

Mix well applesauce, sugar, cinnamon, milk and eggs in a mixing bowl.

One slice at a time, soak the bread into applesauce mixture until wet.

On medium fire, heat a large nonstick skillet.

Add soaked bread on one side and another on the other side. Cook in a single layer in batches for 2-3 minutes per side on medium low fire or until lightly browned.

Serve and enjoy.

Nutrition:

Calories: 122.6,

Fat: 2.6 g

Carbs: 18.3 g

Protein: 6.5 g

Sugars: 14.8 g

Sodium: 11%

Banana-Peanut Butter 'n Greens Smoothie

Preparation time: 5 mins

Cooking time: 0 mins

Servings: 1

Ingredients:

1 c. chopped and packed Romaine lettuce

1 frozen medium banana

1 tbsp. all-natural peanut butter

1 c. cold almond milk

Directions:

In a heavy-duty blender, add all ingredients.

Puree until smooth and creamy.

Serve and enjoy.

Nutrition:

Calories: 349.3, Fat:9.7 g

Carbs:57.4 g Protein:8.1 g

Sugars:4.3 g Sodium:18%

Baking Powder Biscuits

Preparation time: 5 mins

Cooking time: 5 mins

Servings: 1

Ingredients:

1 egg white

1 c. white whole-wheat flour

4 tbsps. Non-hydrogenated vegetable shortening

1 tbsp. sugar

2/3 c. low-

Fat milk

1 c. unbleached all-purpose flour

4 tsps.

Sodium-free baking powder

Directions:

Preheat oven to 450°F. Take out a baking sheet and set aside.

Place the flour, sugar, and baking powder into a mixing bowl and whisk well to combine.

Cut the shortening into the mixture using your fingers, and work until it resembles coarse crumbs. Add the egg white and milk and stir to combine.

Turn the dough out onto a lightly floured surface and knead 1 minute. Roll dough to ¾ inch thickness and cut into 12 rounds.

Place rounds on the baking sheet. Place baking sheet on middle rack in oven and bake 10 minutes.

Remove baking sheet and place biscuits on a wire rack to cool.

Nutrition: Calories: 118, Fat:4 g Carbs:16 g

Protein:3 g Sugars:0.2 g Sodium: 6%

Oatmeal Banana Pancakes with Walnuts

Preparation time: 15 mins

Cooking time: 5 mins

Servings: 8 pancakes

Ingredients:

1 finely diced firm banana

1 c. whole wheat pancake mix

1/8 c. chopped walnuts

¼ c. old-fashioned oats

Directions:

Make the pancake mix according to the directions on the package.

Add walnuts, oats, and chopped banana.

Coat a griddle with cooking spray. Add about ¼ cup of the pancake batter onto the griddle when hot.

Turn pancake over when bubbles form on top. Cook until golden brown.

Serve immediately.

Nutrition:

Calories: 155

Fat: 4 g

Carbs: 28 g

Protein: 7 g

Sugars: 2.2 g

Sodium: 16%

Creamy Oats, Greens & Blueberry Smoothie

Preparation time: 4 mins

Cooking time: 0 mins

Servings: 1

Ingredients:

1 c. cold

Fat-free milk

1 c. salad greens

½ c. fresh frozen blueberries

½ c. frozen cooked oatmeal

1 tbsp. sunflower seeds

Directions:

In a powerful blender, blend all ingredients until smooth and creamy.

Serve and enjoy.

Nutrition: Calories: 280,

Fat:6.8 g Carbs:44.0 g

Protein:14.0 g Sugars:32 g

Sodium:141%

Banana & Cinnamon Oatmeal

Preparation time: 5 mins

Cooking time: 0 mins

Servings: 6

Ingredients: 2 c. quick-cooking oats

4 c. Fat-free milk

1 tsp. ground cinnamon

2 chopped large ripe banana

4 tsps. Brown sugar

Extra ground cinnamon

Directions:

Place milk in a skillet and bring to boil. Add oats and cook over medium heat until thickened, for two to four minutes. Stir intermittently.

Add cinnamon, brown sugar and banana and stir to combine.

If you want, serve with the extra cinnamon and milk.   Enjoy!

Nutrition: Calories: 215, Fat:2 g Carbs:42 g

Protein:10 g Sugars:1 g Sodium:40%

Bagels Made Healthy

Preparation time: 5 mins

Cooking time: 40 mins

Servings: 8

Ingredients:

1 ½ c. warm water

1 ¼ c. bread flour

2 tbsps. Honey

2 c. whole wheat flour

2 tsps. Yeast

1 ½ tbsps. Olive oil

1 tbsp. vinegar

Directions:

In a bread machine, mix all ingredients, and then process on dough cycle.

Once done, create 8 pieces shaped like a flattened ball.

Make a hole in the center of each ball using your thumb then create a donut shape.

In a greased baking sheet, place donut-shaped dough then cover and let it rise about ½ hour.

Prepare about 2 inches of water to boil in a large pan.

In a boiling water, drop one at a time the bagels and boil for 1 minute, then turn them once.

Remove them and return to baking sheet and bake at 350oF for about 20 to 25 minutes until golden brown.

Nutrition:

Calories: 228.1,

Fat:3.7 g

Carbs:41.8 g

Protein:6.9 g

Sugars:0 g

Sodium:15%

Cereal with Cranberry-Orange Twist

Preparation time: 5 mins

Cooking time: 0 mins

Servings: 1

Ingredients:

½ c. water

½ c. orange juice

1/3 c. oat bran

¼ c. dried cranberries

Sugar

Milk

Directions:

In a bowl, combine all ingredients.

For about 2 minutes, microwave the bowl then serve with sugar and milk.

Enjoy!

Nutrition:

Calories: 220.4,

Fat:2.4 g

Carbs:43.5 g

Protein:6.2 g

Sugars:8 g

Sodium:1%

No Cook Overnight Oats

Preparation time: 5 mins

Cooking time: 0 mins

Servings: 1

Ingredients:

1 ½ c. low Fat milk

5 whole almond pieces

1 tsp. chia seeds

2 tbsps. Oats

1 tsp. sunflower seeds

1 tbsp. Craisins

Directions:

In a jar or mason bottle with cap, mix all ingredients.

Refrigerate overnight.

Enjoy for breakfast. Will keep in the fridge for up to 3 days.

Nutrition: Calories: 271,   Fat:9.8 g
Carbs:35.4 g Protein:16.7 g

Sugars:9 Sodium:103%

Avocado Cup with Egg

Preparation time: 5 mins

Cooking time: 0 mins

Servings: 4

Ingredients:

4 tsps. parmesan cheese

1 chopped stalk scallion

4 dashes pepper

4 dashes paprika

2 ripe avocados

4 medium eggs

Directions:

Preheat oven to 375 0F.

Slice avocadoes in half and discard seed.

Slice the rounded portions of the avocado, to make it level and sit well on a baking sheet.

Place avocadoes on baking sheet and crack one egg in each hole of the avocado.

Season each egg evenly with pepper, and paprika.

Pop in the oven and bake for 25 minutes or until eggs are cooked to your liking.

Serve with a sprinkle of parmesan.

Nutrition:

Calories: 206,

Fat:15.4 g Carbs:11.3 g

Protein:8.5 g Sugars:0.4 g

Sodium:21%

Mediterranean Toast

Preparation time: 10 mins

Servings: 2

Cooking time: 0 mins

Ingredients:

1 ½ tsp. reduced-Fat crumbled feta

3 sliced Greek olives

¼ mashed avocado

1 slice good whole wheat bread

1 tbsp. roasted red pepper hummus

3 sliced cherry tomatoes

1 sliced hardboiled egg

Directions:

First, toast the bread and top it with ¼ mashed avocado and 1 tablespoon hummus.

Add the cherry tomatoes, olives, hardboiled egg and feta.

To taste, season with salt and pepper.

Nutrition:

Calories: 333.7,

Fat:17 g

Carbs:33.3 g

Protein:16.3 g

Sugars:1 g

Sodium:19%

Instant Banana Oatmeal

Preparation time: 1 min

Servings: 1

Cooking time: 0 mins

Ingredients:

1 mashed ripe banana

½ c. water

½ c. quick oats

Directions:

Measure the oats and water into a microwave-safe bowl and stir to combine.

Place bowl in microwave and heat on high for 2 minutes.

Remove bowl from microwave and stir in the mashed banana and enjoy.

Nutrition:

Calories: 243

Fat: 3 g

Carbs: 50 g

Protein: 6 g

Sugars: 20 g

Sodium: 30 mg

Almond Butter-Banana Smoothie

Preparation time: 5 mins

Servings: 1

Cooking time: 0 mins

Ingredients:

1 tbsp. almond butter

½ c. ice cubes

½ c. packed spinach

1 peeled and frozen medium banana

1 c.

Fat-free milk

Directions:

In a powerful blender, blend all ingredients until smooth and creamy.

Serve and enjoy.

Nutrition:

Calories: 293,

Fat:9.8 g

Carbs:42.5 g

Protein:13.5 g

Sugars:12 g

Sodium:40%

Brown Sugar Cinnamon Oatmeal

Preparation time: 1 min

Servings: 4

Cooking time: 0 mins

Ingredients: ½ tsp. ground cinnamon

1 ½ tsps. pure vanilla extract

¼ c. light brown sugar 2 c. low-

Fat milk

1 1/3 c. quick oats

Directions:

Measure the milk and vanilla into a medium saucepan and bring to a boil over medium-high heat.

Once boiling reduce heat to medium. Stir in oats, brown sugar, and cinnamon, and cook, stirring2–3 minutes.

Serve immediately, sprinkled with additional cinnamon if desired.

Nutrition: Calories: 208

Fat:3 g

Carbs:38 g

Protein:8 g

Sugars:15 g

Sodium:33%

Buckwheat Pancakes with Vanilla Almond Milk

Preparation time: 10 mins

Servings: 1

Cooking time: 10 mins

Ingredients:

½ c. unsweetened vanilla almond milk

2-4 packets natural sweetener

1/8 tsp. salt

½ cup buckwheat flour

½ tsp. double-acting baking powder

Directions:

Prepare a nonstick pancake griddle and spray with the cooking spray, place over medium heat.

Whisk together the buckwheat flour, salt, baking powder, and stevia in a small bowl and stir in the almond milk after.

Onto the pan, scoop a large spoonful of batter, cook until bubbles no longer pop on the surface and the entire surface looks dry and (2-4 minutes). Flip and cook for another 2-4 minutes. Repeat with all the remaining batter.

Nutrition:

Calories: 240,

Fat:4.5 g

Carbs:2 g

Protein:11 g

Sugars:17 g

Sodium:38%

Tomato Bruschetta with Basil

Preparation time: 10 mins

Servings: 8

Cooking time: 10 mins

Ingredients:

½ c. chopped basil

2 minced garlic cloves

1 tbsp. balsamic vinegar

2 tbsps. Olive oil

½ tsp. cracked black pepper

1 sliced whole wheat baguette

8 diced ripe Roma tomatoes

1 tsp. sea salt

Directions:

First, preheat the oven to 375 F.

In a bowl, dice the tomatoes, mix in balsamic vinegar, chopped basil, garlic, salt, pepper, and olive oil, set aside.

Slice the baguette into 16-18 slices and for about 10 minutes, place on a baking pan to bake.

Serve with warm bread slices and enjoy.

For leftovers, store in an airtight container and put in the fridge. Try putting them over grilled chicken, it is amazing!

Nutrition:

Calories: 57, Fat:2.5 g Carbs:7.9 g

Protein:1.4 g Sugars:0.2 g Sodium:12%

Sweet Corn Muffins

Preparation time: 5 mins

Servings: 1

Cooking time: 10 mins

Ingredients:

1 tbsp. Sodium-free baking powder

¾ c. nondairy milk

1 tsp. pure vanilla extract

½ c. sugar

1 c. white whole-wheat flour

1 c. cornmeal

½ c. canola oil

Directions:

Preheat the oven to 400°F. Line a 12-muffin tin with paper liners and set aside.

Place the cornmeal, flour, sugar, and baking powder into a mixing bowl and whisk well to combine.

Add the nondairy milk, oil, and vanilla and stir just until combined.

Divide the batter evenly between the muffin cups. Place muffin tin on middle rack in oven and bake for 15 minutes.

Remove from oven and place on a wire rack to cool.

Nutrition: Calories: 203,

Fat:9 g Carbs:26 g Protein:3 g

Sugars:9.5 g Sodium:8%

Scrambled Eggs with Mushrooms and Spinach

Preparation time: 5 mins

Servings: 1

Cooking time: 10 mins

Ingredients: 2 egg whites

1 slice whole wheat toast

½ c. sliced fresh mushrooms

2 tbsps. Shredded

Fat free American cheese

Pepper

1 tsp. olive oil

1 c. chopped fresh spinach

1 whole egg

Directions:

On medium high fire, place a nonstick fry pan and add oil. Swirl oil to cover pan and heat for a minute.

Add spinach and mushrooms. Sauté until spinach is wilted, around 2-3 minutes.

Meanwhile, in a bowl whisk well egg whites, and cheese. Season with pepper.

Pour egg mixture into pan and scramble until eggs are cooked through, around 3-4 minutes.

Serve and enjoy with a piece of whole wheat toast.

Nutrition:

Calories: 290.6, Fat:11.8 g Carbs:21.8 g

Protein:24.3 g Sugars:1.4 g Sodium:24%

Chia and Oat Breakfast Bran

Preparation time: overnight

Servings: 2

Cooking time: 0 mins

Ingredients:

85 g chopped roasted almonds

340 g coconut milk

30 g cane sugar

2½ g orange zest

30 g flax seed mix

170 g rolled oats

340 g blueberries

30 g chia seeds

2½ g cinnamon

Directions:

Add all your wet ingredients together and mix the sugar and milk in with the orange zest.

Stir in the cinnamon and mix well. Once you are sure the sugar isn't lumpy add in the rolled oats, flax seeds, and chia and then let it sit for a minute.

Grab two bowls or mason jars and pour the mixture in. Top with the roasted almonds, and store in the fridge.

Pull it out in the morning and dig in!

Nutrition:

Calories: 353, Fat:8 g Carbs:55 g

Protein:15 g Sugars:9.9 g Sodium:26%

7 ½ g garlic powder

2 ½ g pepper

170 g shredded low-Fat cheese

170 g grated sweet potato

2 ½ g salt

Directions:

Preheat oven to 400 0F and prepare a muffin tin with liners.

Place grated sweet potatoes, onions, garlic, and spices into a bowl and mix well, before placing one spoonful in each cup. Add one large egg upon each cup and proceed to bake for 15 minutes until eggs are cooked.

Serve fresh or store.

Nutrition:

Calories: 143,

Fat:9.1 g

Carbs:6 g

Protein:9 g Sugars:0 g

Sodium:11%

Faux Breakfast Hash Brown Cups

Preparation time: 15 mins

Servings: 8

Cooking time: 0 mins

Ingredients:

40 g diced onion

8 large eggs

Maple Mocha Frappe

Preparation time: 2 mins

Servings: 2

Cooking time: 0 mins

Ingredients:

1 tbsp. unsweetened cocoa powder

½ c. low-

Fat milk

2 tbsps. Pure maple syrup

½ c. brewed coffee

1 small ripe banana

1 c. low-

Fat vanilla yogurt

Directions:

Place the banana in a blender or food processor and purée.

Add the remaining ingredients and pulse until smooth and creamy.

Serve immediately.

Nutrition: Calories: 206, Fat:2 g Carbs:38 g

Protein:6 g Sugars:17 g Sodium:23%

Breakfast Oatmeal in Slow Cooker

Preparation time: 10 mins

Servings: 8

Cooking time: 8 hours

Ingredients: 4 c. almond milk

2 packets stevia   2 c. steel-cut oats

1/3 c. chopped dried apricots 4 c. water

1/3 c. dried cherries   1 tsp. cinnamon

1/3 c. raisins

Directions:

In slow cooker, mix well all ingredients.

Cover and set to low.

Cook for 8 hours.

You can set this the night before so that by morning you have breakfast ready.

Nutrition: Calories: 158.5, Fat:2.9 g

Carbs:28.3 g Protein:4.8 g Sugars:11 g

Sodium:48%

Apple Cinnamon Overnight Oats

Preparation time: 15 mins

Servings: 2

Cooking time: 0 mins

Ingredients:

1 diced apple

2 tbsps. Chia seeds

½ tbsp. ground cinnamon

½ tsp. pure vanilla extract

1¼ c. non

Fat milk

Kosher salt

1 c. old-fashioned rolled oats

2 tsps. Honey

Directions:

Divide the oats, chia seeds or ground flaxseed, milk, cinnamon, honey or maple syrup, vanilla extract, and salt into two Mason jars. Place the lids tightly on top and shake until thoroughly combined.

Remove the lids and add half of the diced apple to each jar. Sprinkle with additional cinnamon, if desired. Place the lids tightly back on the jars and refrigerate for at least 4 hours or overnight.

You can store the overnight oats in single-serve containers in the refrigerator for up to 3 days.

Nutrition: Calories: 339,

Fat:8 g Carbs:60 g Protein:13 g

Sugars:15 g

Sodium:11%

Spinach Mushroom Omelette

Preparation time: 5 mins

Servings: 2

Cooking time: 5 mins

Ingredients:

2 tbsps. Olive oil

2 whole eggs

3 c. spinach, fresh

Cooking spray

10 sliced baby Bella mushrooms

8 tbsps. Sliced red onion

4 egg whites

2 oz. goat cheese

Directions:

Place a skillet over medium-high heat and add olive.

Add the sliced red onions to the pan and stir until translucent. Then, add your mushrooms to the pan and keep stirring until they are slightly brown.

Add spinach and stir until they wilted. Season with a tiny bit of pepper and salt. Remove from heat.

Spray a small pan with cooking spray and Place over medium heat.

Break 2 whole eggs in a small bowl. Add 4 egg whites and whisk to combine.

Pour the whisked eggs into the small skillet and allow the mixture to sit for a minute.

Use a spatula to gently work your way around the skillet's edges. Raise the skillet and tip it down and around in a circular style to allow the runny eggs to reach the center and cook around the edges of the skillet.

Add crumbled goat cheese to a side of the omelet top with your mushroom mixture.

Then, gently fold the other side of the omelet over the mushroom side with the spatula.

1Allowing cooking for thirty seconds. Then, transfer the omelet to a plate.

Nutrition: Calories: 412,

Fat:29 g Carbs:18 g Protein:25 g

Sugars:7 g Sodium:49%

Muesli Scones

Preparation time: 10 minutes

Cook time: 15 minutes

Servings: 16

Ingredients:

1 egg;

1/4 cup dried cranberries;

1/4 cup dried apricots, chopped;

1/4 cup pistachios, coarsely chopped;

1/4 cup sunflower seeds;

1/4 cup raw sesame seeds;

2 tablespoons agave nectar or honey;

2 cups blanched almond flour (not almond meal);

1/2 teaspoon baking soda.

Instructions:

1. Combine almond flour and soda in a bowl.

2. Then add dried fruit, seeds, and nuts.

3. Combine egg and agave in a bowl.

4. Combine egg/agave mixture with the flour/dried fruit mixture and form the dough with your hands.

5. Shape the dough into a 6.5*6.5-inch square that is about 3/4-inch thick and divide it into 16 squares.

6. Heat the oven to 350 °F. Put dough squares on a baking sheet lined with parchment paper and bake for 10-12 minutes.

Nutritional info (per serving): 76 calories; 5.7 g

Fat; 5.0 g carbohydrate; 2.6 g

Protein; 106 mg

Sodium; 9%

Fiber.

Sweet Potato Waffles

Preparation time: 5 minutes

Cook time: 10 minutes

Servings: 6

Ingredients:

1/2 cup sweet potato;

1 cup oats;

2 eggs;

1 cup almond milk;

1 tablespoon honey;

maple syrup;

banana, sliced;

1/4 teaspoon baking powder;

1 tablespoon olive oil.

Instructions:

1. Combine all ingredients in a blender jar. Blend them until fully pureed.

2. Heat the waffle iron and spray it with cooking spray.

3. Pour 1/3 cup of batter into each waffle mold and cook for 3-4 minutes.

4. Once cooked, serve with maple syrup and fresh, chopped banana.

Nutritional info (per serving): 237 calories; 14.3 g

Fat; 24.6 g carbohydrate; 5.1 g

Protein; 131 mg

Sodium; 3.3 g

Fiber.

Ezekiel Bread French Toast

Preparation time: 5 minutes

Cook time: 15 minutes

Servings: 2

Ingredients:

4 slices of Ezekiel bread;

1/2 cup coconut milk or unsweetened almond milk;

2 eggs;

2 tablespoons coconut sugar;

1 teaspoon vanilla;

1 packet stevia;

cinnamon.

Instructions:

1. Combine every ingredient (except for the Ezekiel bread) in a bowl.

2. Fully dip each slice of bread into the mixture.

3. Cook in a skillet for about 4 minutes on each side, or until lightly browned.

4. Once cooked, serve with syrup.

Nutritional info (per serving): 461 calories; 18.7 g

Fat; 58.9 g carbohydrate; 13.9 g

Protein; 241 mg

Sodium; 41%

Fiber.

Mushroom Spinach Omelet

Preparation time: 3 minutes

Cook time: 15 minutes

Servings: 2

Ingredients: 1 tablespoon olive oil;

1/4 cup red onion, sliced;

green onions, diced; 1 oz. goat cheese;

1.5 cups fresh spinach;

5 baby bella mushrooms, sliced;

1 whole egg; 2 egg whites;

garlic powder, black pepper, to taste.

Instructions:

1. Heat oil in a medium skillet on medium-high heat.

2. Add red onions and sauté for 2-3 minutes. Add sliced mushrooms and sauté for 4-5 minutes.

3. Add spinach, sauté for about 2 minutes and season with garlic powder and pepper. Then set aside.

4. Whisk eggs in a bowl. Pour the egg mixture into a small skillet and cook it on medium heat till eggs are no longer runny.

5. Put mushroom/spinach mixture on top of the omelet and sprinkle it with goat cheese.

6. Fold omelet in half and cook for another 30 seconds. Once cooked, put omelet onto a plate and top with green onions.

Nutritional info (per serving): 412 calories; 29.2 g

Fat; 18.1 g carbohydrate; 25.2 g

Protein; 332 mg

Sodium; 25% Fiber.

Chapter 5 Lunch recipes

Veggie Quesadillas

Preparation time: 10 minutes

Cooking time: 4 minutes

Servings: 3

Ingredients:

1 cup black beans, cooked

½ red bell pepper, chopped

4 tablespoons cilantro, chopped

½ cup corn

1 cup low-

Fat cheddar, shredded

6 whole wheat tortillas

1 carrot, shredded

1 small jalapeno pepper, chopped

1 cup non-

Fat yogurt

Juice of ½ lime

Directions:

Divide black beans, red bell pepper, 2 tablespoons cilantro, corn, carrot, jalapeno and the cheese on half of the tortillas and cover with the other ones.

Heat up a pan over medium-high heat, add one quesadilla, cook for 3 minutes on one side, flip, cook for 1 more minute on the other and transfer to a plate.

Repeat with the rest of the quesadillas.

In a bowl, combine 2 tablespoons cilantro with yogurt and lime juice, whisk well and serve next to the quesadillas.

Enjoy!

Nutrition:

calories 200,

Fat 3,

Fiber 4,

Carbs 13,

Protein 7

Sodium 94%

Chicken Wraps

Preparation time: 10 minutes

Cooking time: 10 minutes

Servings: 4

Ingredients:

8 ounces chicken breast, cubed

½ cup celery, chopped

2/3 cup mandarin oranges, chopped

¼ cup onion, chopped

A drizzle of olive oil

2 tablespoons mayonnaise

¼ teaspoon garlic powder

A pinch of black pepper

4 whole wheat tortillas

4 lettuce leaves

Directions:

Heat up a pan with the oil over medium-high heat, add chicken cubes, cook for 5 minutes on each side and transfer to a bowl.

Divide the chicken on each tortilla, also divide celery, oranges, onion, mayo, garlic powder, black pepper and lettuce leaves, wrap and serve for lunch.

Enjoy!

Nutrition:

calories 200,

Fat 3,

Fiber 4,

Carbs 13,

Protein 7

Sodium 84%

Black Bean Patties with Cilantro

Preparation time: 10 minutes

Cooking time: 10 minutes

Servings: 4

Ingredients:

2 whole wheat bread slices, torn

3 tablespoons cilantro, chopped

2 garlic cloves, minced

15 ounces canned black beans, no-salt-added, drained and rinsed

6 ounces canned chipotle peppers, chopped

1 teaspoon cumin, ground

1 egg

Cooking spray

½ avocado, peeled, pitted and mashed

1 tablespoon lime juice

1 cherry tomato, chopped

Directions:

Put the bread in your food processor, pulse well and transfer bread crumbs to a bowl.

Combine them with cilantro, garlic, black beans, chipotle peppers, cumin and egg stir well and shape 4 patties out of this mix.

Heat up a pan over medium-high heat, grease with cooking spray, add beans patties, cook them for 5 minutes on each side and transfer to plates.

In a bowl, combine the avocado with tomato and lime juice, stir well, add over the patties and serve for lunch.

Enjoy!

Nutrition:

calories 200,

Fat 4,

Fiber 4,

Carbs 12,

Protein 8

Sodium 2%

Lunch Rice Bowls

Preparation time: 10 minutes

Cooking time: 5 minutes

Servings: 2

Ingredients:

1 teaspoon olive oil

1 cup mixed bell peppers, onion, zucchini and corn, chopped

1 cup chicken meat, cooked and shredded

1 cup brown rice, cooked

3 tablespoons salsa

2 tablespoons low-

Fat cheddar, shredded

2 tablespoons low-

Fat sour cream

Directions:

Heat up a pan with the oil over medium-high heat, add mixed veggies, stir and cook them for 5 minutes.

Divide the rice and the chicken meat into 2 bowls, add mixed veggies and top each with salsa, cheese and sour cream.

Serve for lunch.

Enjoy!

Nutrition:

calories 199

Fat 4,

Fiber 4,

Carbs 12,

Protein 7

Sodium 85%

Salmon Salad

Preparation time: 10 minutes

Cooking time: 0 minutes

Servings: 3

Ingredients: 1 cup canned salmon, flaked

1 tablespoon lemon juice 3 tablespoons

Fat-free yogurt

2 tablespoons red bell pepper, chopped

1 teaspoon capers, drained and chopped

1 tablespoon red onion, chopped

1 teaspoon dill, chopped

A pinch of black pepper

3 whole wheat bread slices

Directions:

In a bowl, combine the salmon with the lemon juice, yogurt, bell pepper, capers, onion, dill and black pepper and stir well.

Spread this on each bread slice and serve for lunch. Enjoy!

Nutrition:

Calories: 199

Fat: 2

Fiber: 4

Carbs: 14

Protein: 8

Sodium: 45%

Stuffed Mushrooms Caps

Preparation time: 10 minutes

Cooking time: 15 minutes

Servings: 2

Ingredients:

2 Portobello mushroom caps

2 tablespoons pesto

2 tomato, chopped

¼ cup low-

Fat mozzarella, shredded

Directions:

Divide pesto, tomato and mozzarella in each mushroom cap, arrange them on a lined baking sheet, introduce in the oven and bake at 400 degrees F for 15 minutes.

Serve for lunch. Enjoy!

Nutrition: calories 198, Fat 3,

Fiber 4, Carbs 14,

Protein 9 Sodium 19%

Tuna Salad

Preparation time: 10 minutes

Cooking time: 0 minutes

Servings: 3

Ingredients:

5 ounces canned tuna in water, drained

1 tablespoon red vinegar

1 tablespoon olive oil

¼ cup green onions, chopped

2 cups arugula 1 tablespoon low-

Fat parmesan, grated

A pinch of black pepper

2 ounces whole wheat pasta, cooked

Directions: In a bowl, combine the tuna with the vinegar, oil, green onions, arugula, pasta and black pepper and toss.

Divide between 3 plates, sprinkle parmesan on top and serve for lunch. Enjoy!

Nutrition:

Calories: 200

Fat: 4

Fiber: 4

Carbs: 14

Protein: 7

Sodium: 2%

Shrimp Lunch Rolls

Preparation time: 10 minutes

Cooking time: 0 minutes

Servings: 4

Ingredients:

12 rice paper sheets, soaked for a few seconds in warm water and drained

1 cup cilantro, chopped

12 basil leaves

12 baby lettuce leaves

1 small cucumber, sliced

1 cup carrots, shredded

20 ounces shrimp, cooked, peeled and deveined

Directions:

Arrange all rice papers on a working surface, divide cilantro, bay leaves, baby lettuce leaves, cucumber, carrots and shrimp, wrap, seal edges and serve for lunch. Enjoy!

Nutrition: calories 200, Fat 4, Fiber 4,

Carbs 14, Protein 8 Sodium 100%

Turkey Sandwich with Mozzarella

Preparation time: 10 minutes

Cooking time: 3 minutes

Servings: 2

Ingredients:

2 whole wheat bread slices

2 teaspoons mustard

2 sliced smoked turkey

1 pear, cored and sliced

¼ cup low-Fat mozzarella, shredded

Directions:

Spread the mustard on each bread slice, divide turkey slices on one bread slice, add pear slices and mozzarella, top with the other bread slice, introduce in preheated broiler for 3 minutes, cut the sand which in halves and serve. Enjoy!

Nutrition: calories 171, Fat 2, Fiber 4,

Carbs 9, Protein 9

Sodium 16%

Veggie Soup

Preparation time: 10 minutes

Cooking time: 16 minutes

Servings: 6

Ingredients:

2 teaspoons olive oil

1 and ½ cups carrot, shredded

6 garlic cloves, minced

1 cup yellow onion, chopped

1 cup celery, chopped

32 ounces low-

Sodium chicken stock

4 cups water

1 and ½ cups whole wheat pasta

2 tablespoons parsley, chopped

¼ cup low-

Fat parmesan, grated

Directions:

Heat up a pot with the oil over medium-high heat, add garlic, stir and cook for 1 minute.

Add onion, carrot and celery, stir and cook for 7 minutes.

Add stock, water and pasta, stir, bring to a boil over medium heat and cook for 8 minutes more.

Divide into bowls, top each with parsley and parmesan and serve. Enjoy!

Nutrition: calories 212, Fat 4,

Fiber 4, Carbs 13, Protein 8 Sodium 17%

Avocado and Melon Salad

Preparation time: 10 minutes

Cooking time: 0 minutes

Servings: 4

Ingredients:

2 tablespoons stevia

2 tablespoon red vinegar

2 tablespoons mint, chopped

A pinch of black pepper

1 avocado, peeled, pitted and sliced

4 cups baby spinach

½ small cantaloupe, peeled and cubed

1 and ½ cups strawberries, sliced

2 teaspoons sesame seeds, toasted

Directions:

In a salad bowl, combine the avocado with baby spinach, cantaloupe and strawberries and toss.

In another bowl, combine the stevia with vinegar, mint and black pepper, whisk, add to your salad, toss, sprinkle sesame seeds on top and serve.

Enjoy!

Nutrition: calories 199,

Fat 3, Fiber 4,

Carbs 12, Protein 8

Sodium 5%

Spaghetti Squash And Sauce

Preparation time: 10 minutes

Cooking time: 25 minutes

Servings: 4

Ingredients:

1 pound beef, ground

½ cup yellow onion, chopped

½ cup green bell pepper, chopped

2 garlic cloves, minced

14 ounces canned tomatoes, no-salt-added, chopped

2 tablespoons tomato paste

8 ounces tomato sauce

1 teaspoon Italian seasoning

¼ cup low-

Fat parmesan, shredded

2 pounds spaghetti squash, pricked with a knife

Directions:

Put the spaghetti squash on a lined baking sheet, introduce in the oven, bake at 400 degrees F for 10 minutes, cut into halves, shred and separate squash pulp into spaghetti and put into a bowl.

Heat up a pan over medium-high heat, add the beef, stir and brown for 5 minutes.

Add onion, bell pepper, garlic, tomatoes, tomato paste, tomato sauce and Italian seasoning stir and cook for 10 minutes.

Divide the squash spaghetti between plates, top each with beef mix, sprinkle parmesan on top and serve. Enjoy!

Nutrition: calories 231, Fat 4,

Fiber 5, Carbs 14, Protein 9

Sodium 24%

Sausage with Potatoes

Preparation time: 10 minutes

Cooking time: 22 minutes

Servings: 6

Ingredients:

½ pound smoked sausage, cooked and chopped

3 tablespoons olive oil

1 and ¾ pounds red potatoes, cubed

2 yellow onions, chopped

1 teaspoon thyme, dried

2 teaspoons cumin, ground

A pinch of black pepper

Directions:

Heat up a pan with the oil over medium-high heat, add potatoes and onions, stir and cook for 12 minutes. Add sausage, thyme, cumin and black pepper, stir, cook for 10 minutes more, divide between plates and serve for lunch. Enjoy!

Nutrition: calories 199, Fat 2, Fiber 4,

Carbs 14, Protein 8 Sodium 24%

Beef Soup

Preparation time: 10 minutes

Cooking time: 20 minutes

Servings: 4

Ingredients:

1 tablespoon olive oil

1 yellow onion, chopped

1 pound beef sirloin, ground

32 ounces low-

Sodium beef stock

1/3 cup whole wheat flour

1 pound mixed carrots and celery, chopped

Directions:

Heat up a pot with the oil over medium-high heat, add beef and flour, stir well and brown for 5 minutes.

Add onion, carrots, celery and stock, stir, bring to a simmer, reduce heat to medium, cook the soup for 15 minutes, ladle into bowls and serve for lunch.

Enjoy!

Nutrition:

calories 281,

Fat 3,

Fiber 5,

Carbs 14,

Protein 11

Sodium 11%

Shrimp Salad

Preparation time: 10 minutes

Cooking time: 8 minutes

Servings: 4

Ingredients:

12 ounces asparagus spears, trimmed and halved

8 ounces baby corn

12 endive leaves, torn

12 baby lettuce leaves

12 spinach leaves

12 ounces shrimp, cooked, peeled and deveined

2 and ½ cups red raspberries

¼ cup olive oil

¼ cup raspberry vinegar

1 tablespoon cilantro, chopped

2 teaspoons stevia

Directions:

Put some water in a pot, bring to a boil over medium-high heat, add asparagus, cook for 8 minutes, transfer to a bowl filled with ice water, cool down, drain well and put in a salad bowl. Add corn, endive leaves, spinach, lettuce, shrimp and raspberries.

In another bowl, combine the oil with the vinegar, stevia and cilantro, whisk well, add to your salad, toss and serve for lunch. Enjoy!

Nutrition: calories 199, Fat 2, Fiber 3,

Carbs 14, Protein 8 Sodium 54%

Watercress, Asparagus And Shrimp Salad

Preparation time: 10 minutes

Cooking time: 4 minutes

Servings: 4

Ingredients:

12 ounces asparagus spears, trimmed

16 ounces shrimp, cooked, peeled and deveined

4 cups watercress, torn

2 cups cherry tomatoes, halved

¼ cup raspberry vinegar ¼ cup olive oil

Directions:

Put the asparagus in a pot, add water to cover, cook over medium heat for 4 minutes, drain, transfer to a bowl filled with ice water, cool down, drain again and transfer to a salad bowl. Add shrimp, watercress, tomatoes, raspberry vinegar and oil, toss well and serve for lunch. Enjoy!

Nutrition: calories 212, Fat 4, Fiber 7,

Carbs 14, Protein 9 Sodium 74%

Chicken Tacos

Preparation time: 10 minutes

Cooking time: 0 minutes

Servings: 2

Ingredients: 4 mini taco shells

2 tablespoons celery, chopped

1 tablespoon light mayonnaise

1 tablespoon salsa 1 tablespoon low-

Fat cheddar, shredded

1/3 cup chicken, cooked and shredded

Directions:

In a bowl, combine the celery with the mayo, salsa, cheddar and chicken and toss well.

Spoon this into mini taco shells and serve for lunch. Enjoy!

Nutrition: calories 221, Fat 3,

Fiber 8, Carbs 14, Protein 9 Sodium 48%

Millet Cakes

Preparation time: 10 minutes

Cooking time: 55 minutes

Servings: 4

Ingredients:

1 tablespoon olive oil 1 cup millet

¼ cup yellow onion, chopped

1 garlic clove, minced

3 and ½ cups water

A pinch of black pepper

1/3 cup zucchini, shredded

1/3 cup carrot, shredded 1/3 cup low-

Fat parmesan, grated

1 and ½ teaspoon thyme, chopped

1 teaspoon lemon zest, grated

Cooking spray

Directions:

Heat up a pan with 1 tablespoon olive oil over medium heat, add onion, stir and cook for 4 minutes.

Add garlic and millet, stir and cook for 1 more minute.

Add the water and a pinch of black pepper, stir, cover, reduce heat to low and cook for 20 minutes stirring once.

Add carrot, zucchini, thyme, parmesan and lemon zest, stir and cook for 10 minutes more.

Leave the millet mix to cool down, shape 12 millet cakes using damp hands and put them on a working surface.

Heat up a pan with cooking spray over medium-high heat, add millet cakes, cook them for 5 minutes on each side, divide them between plates and serve.

Enjoy!

Nutrition: calories 211, Fat 4,

Fiber 4, Carbs 14,

Protein 6 Sodium 6%

Lentils Dal with Yogurt

Preparation time: 10 minutes

Cooking time: 10 minutes

Servings: 4

Ingredients:

1 and ½ teaspoons olive oil

1 yellow onion, chopped

2 teaspoons curry powder

14 ounces canned lentils, no-salt-added, drained and rinsed

14 ounces canned tomatoes, chopped

2 pounds chicken, roasted, and chopped

A pinch of black pepper

¼ cup low-

Fat yogurt

Directions:

Heat up a pot with the oil over medium-high heat, add onion, stir and brown for 4 minutes.

Add curry powder, stir and cook for 1 more minute.

Add lentils, tomatoes, chicken and black pepper, stir, cook for 5 minutes more, take off heat, add the yogurt, toss, divide into bowls and serve for lunch.

Enjoy!

Nutrition:

calories 199,

Fat 3,

Fiber 7,

Carbs 17,

Protein 8

Sodium 21%

Lunch Quinoa And Spinach Salad

Preparation time: 10 minutes

Cooking time: 25 minutes

Servings: 4

Ingredients:

1 cup quinoa 2 teaspoons olive oil

½ cup apricots, dried and chopped

2 garlic cloves, minced

2 cups water A pinch of black pepper

1 cup cherry tomatoes, halved

1 red onion, chopped

8 cups baby spinach

¼ cup almonds, sliced

For the salad dressing:

½ teaspoon lemon zest, grated

2 tablespoons lemon juice

1 teaspoon coconut sugar

½ teaspoon Dijon mustard

4 tablespoons olive oil

Directions:

Heat up a pan over medium heat, add quinoa, toast for 5 minutes and transfer to a bowl.

Heat up a pan with the oil over medium heat, add garlic, stir and cook for 1 minute.

Add quinoa and apricots, stir and cook for 4 minutes more.

Add water, bring to a boil and simmer for 15 minutes more.

In a salad bowl, combine the tomatoes with the onion, spinach, almonds, quinoa and apricots.

In another bowl, combine the lemon zest with the lemon juice, sugar, mustard and oil, whisk well, add to the quinoa salad, toss and serve for lunch. Enjoy!

Nutrition: calories 199, Fat 3, Fiber 4,

Carbs 16, Protein 8 Sodium 4%

Italian Pasta with Parmesan

Preparation time: 10 minutes

Cooking time: 20 minutes

Servings: 4

Ingredients:

1 pound whole wheat penne pasta, cooked

3 garlic cloves, minced

2 tablespoons olive oil 3 carrots, sliced

1 bunch asparagus, trimmed and cut into medium pieces

1 red bell pepper, chopped

1 yellow bell pepper, chopped

1 cup cherry tomatoes, halved

A pinch of black pepper

2/3 cup coconut cream

2 tablespoons low-

Fat parmesan, grated

Directions:

Heat up a pan with the oil over medium-high heat, add the garlic, stir and cook for 2 minutes.

Add carrots, stir and cook for 4 minutes more.

Add asparagus, stir, cover the pan and cook for 8 minutes more.

Add yellow and red bell peppers, stir and cook for 5 minutes.

Add cherry tomatoes, black pepper, cream, parmesan and pasta, toss, divide between plates and serve.

Enjoy!

Nutrition:

calories 221,

Fat 4,

Fiber 4,

Carbs 15,

Protein 9

Sodium 20%

Glazed Ribs

Preparation time: 10 minutes

Cooking time: 1 hour and 20 minutes

Servings: 4

Ingredients:

1 rack pork ribs, ribs separated

1 and ¼ cups tomato sauce

¼ cup white vinegar

3 tablespoons spicy mustard

2 tablespoons coconut sugar

3 tablespoons water

¼ teaspoon hot sauce

1 teaspoon onion powder

Cooking spray

Directions:

Put the ribs in a baking dish, cover with tin foil and bake in the oven at 400 degrees F for 1 hour.

Heat up a pan with the tomato sauce, mustard, sugar, vinegar, water, onion powder and hot sauce, stir, cook for 10 minutes and take off heat.

Baste the ribs with half of this sauce, place them on preheated grill over medium-high heat, grease them with cooking spray, cook for 4 minutes on each side, divide between plates and serve with the rest of the sauce on the side.

Enjoy!

Nutrition:

calories 287,

Fat 5,

Fiber 8,

Carbs 16,

Protein 15

Sodium 72%

Chinese Chicken

Preparation time: 10 minutes ,

Cook Time: 10 minutes

Serves: 4

Ingredients:

5 pounds chicken thighs

½ cup balsamic vinegar

1 teaspoon dried black peppercorns

½ cup coconut aminos

black pepper for taste

4 cloves minced garlic.

Directions:

Within the instant pot, mix chicken with vinegar, aminos, garlic, pepper, and the peppercorns. Mix it together.

Then, cook it on high for 15 minutes.

Divide it, and then serve!

Nutrition: Calories 261,

Fat 7g

Carbs 18gNet

Carbs: 10g

Protein: 8g

Fiber 8g

Sodium 33%

Chicken and Barley

Preparation time: 15 minutes , Cook Time: 35 minutes

Servings: 4

Ingredients:

6 oz. Barley

1 pound chicken thighs

5 chopped carrots

12 oz, water

5 oz. Peas

3 chopped yellow onions

6 oz. Low-

Sodium veggie stock

Black pepper for taste

Directions:

Within the instant pot, mix the stock with the barley and water, and cook on highs for 20 minutes.

Add in onions, carrots, peas, and chicken, and then cook on high once again, natural pressure release.

Add more black pepper for taste, and then serve!

Nutrition: Calories: 261,

Fat: 7g Carbs: 18g Net Carbs: 10g

Protein: 7g Fiber: 8g Sodium 39%

Instant Pot Potato Salad

Preparation time: 5 minutes , Cook Time: 10 minutes

Servings: 2

Ingredients:

6 potatoes, peeled and cubed

4 eggs

1 cup mayonnaise

1 tablespoon dill pickle juice

Salt and pepper for taste

2 cups water

¼ cup chopped onion

2 tablespoons chopped parsley

1 tablespoon muster

Directions:

Take your steamer basket and put it in pressure cooker pot.

Add the water, potatoes, and eggs, and then cook on high pressure for 4 minutes.

When finished, pull the eggs out and let them cool in cold water.

Add the other ingredients together, and then the cooled potatoes and mix it in. you can then dice the eggs and put it in the salad, and then add salt and pepper for taste. Let it chill for an hour if you want that.

Nutrition: Calories: 230,

Fat: 9 g Carbs: 22gNet

Carbs: 15 g Protein: 12 g

Fiber: 7 g. Sodium 117%

Instant Pot Beef Gyros

Preparation time: 10 minutes , Cook Time: 15 minutes

Servings: 6

Ingredients:

2 pounds beef roast, thinly sliced

1 tablespoon dried parsley

1 teaspoon salt

3 cloves minced garlic

1 teaspoon black pepper

1 sliced red onion

4 tablespoons oil of choice

1 teaspoon olive oil

½ cup vegetable broth

1 tablespoon lemon juice

For the Tzatziki sauce:

1 cup plain yogurt

1 clove minced garlic

2 tablespoon fresh dill

½ cup cucumber, peeled, seeded, and chopped finely

Directions:

Turn on instant pot and then add oil to the bottom.

Add meat, seasonings, garlic, and onion to sear and soften the onions.

Pour the lemon juice and broth over meat, and then stir it, lock lid into place, and then use meat/stew and cook it for 9 minutes.

Let it natural release pressure for 3 minutes before quickly released.

Mix the Tzatziki sauce and if you want vegetable toppings or apple cider vinegar over this, you can.

You can also put lettuce at the bottom of naan or pita bread before adding meat and toppings.

Nutrition: Calories: 395,

Fat: 27g

Carbs: 4gNet

Carbs: 4g

Protein: 32g

Fiber: 0g.

Sodium 38%

Instant Pot Lasagna Hamburger Helper

Preparation time: 2 minutes , Cook Time: 5 minutes

Serves: 4

Ingredients: 1 box 16 oz, pasta

8 oz. Ricotta cheese   ½ pound ground beef

1 jar pasta sauce   8 oz. Mozzarella cheese

½ pound ground sausage   4 cups water

Directions:

Put pot in sauté mood and cook meat till brown and crumbled.

Add in rest of ingredients, turn it on high pressure for five minutes.

Quick release it, and then put in half the cheese and half the mozzarella, and then put into a baking pan with more mozzarella. You can cook it for another 2-3 minutes till cheese melts.

Nutrition: Calories: 537, Fat: 33g

Carbs: 25 gNet Carbs: 21g Protein: 34g

Fiber: 4g   Sodium 36%

Pasta with Meat sauce

Preparation time: 10 minutes , Cook Time: 5 minutes

Servings: 4-6

Ingredients: 2 cloves minced garlic

1 diced red pepper   8 oz. Dried pasta

12 oz. Water   1 diced small onion

2 pounds ground meat

1 jar pasta sauce

Directions:

Turn instant pot to sauté setting.

Add in onions, peppers, and meat to cook till no longer pink.

Add pasta, pasta sauce, and water, and stir it.

Set it for 5 minutes manual mode, and then quick release, top with cheese and parsley.

Nutrition: Calories: 437, Fat: 25g

Carbs: 30gNet Carbs: 26g Protein: 24g

Fiber: 4g   Sodium 6%

Tavern Sandwiches in Instant Pot

Preparation time: 5 minutes , Cook Time: 15 minutes

Serves: 8

Ingredients:

2 pounds ground beef

½ teaspoon salt

10 oz. Can chicken gumbo soup with a little bit of liquid left

2 tablespoons mustard

8 slices American cheese

3 chopped green onions

¼ teaspoon pepper

1 can tomato soup

1 tablespoon ketchup

Split sandwich buns

Directions:

Press sauté button on instant pot and cook ground beef till it's not pink.

Add all ingredients but the cheese and bun, cooking it on high for 7 minutes.

Quick release it, and spoon it into a bun, adding cheese to serve.

Nutrition: Calories: 270,

Fat: 10g

Carbs: 22gNet Carbs: 17g

Protein: 20g Fiber: 5g

Sodium 67%

Instant Pot Egg Sandwiches

Preparation time: 5 minutes , Cook Time: 10 minutes

Servings: 2

Ingredients: 2 brown baguettes

6 tab spoons mayonnaise

½ cup spring onion

1 teaspoon mustard powder

Butter, salt, and pepper to taste

6 large eggs   1 large carrot

½ cup cucumbers ½ cup cheese

1 teaspoon parsley

Directions: Put a cup of water at the bottom, and then put eggs in steamer baskets, steaming for 5 minutes.

Prepare your carrot, and dice your cucumber and onion, grate cheese, and add all ingredients but spring onion to the bowl, seasoning this and adding mayonnaise to mix this. Slice the baguettes in half, and when done, remove eggs and put them in cold water, removing shells.

Mash the eggs with the other ingredients till you have an egg mayonnaise, and then sauté the bread as desired with butter until they're browned.

add spring onion and sauté it, and then, layer the bread, mayonnaise mixture, and spring onions, and then serve!

Nutrition: Calories: 260, Fat: 13g

Carbs: 38gNet Carbs: 31g Protein: 33g

Fiber: 7g Sodium 19%

Instant Pot Shredded Chicken

Preparation time: 10 minutes , Cook Time: 16 minutes

Servings: 14

Ingredients:

pounds boneless, skinless chicken breasts

1 teaspoon oregano, dried

½ teaspoon salt

1 cup low-

Sodium chicken broth

½ teaspoon garlic powder

¼ teaspoon black pepper

Directions:

Put chicken within instant pot, then the broth, and rest of the ingredients.

Cook on high pressure for 16 minutes for larger breasts, and then natural pressure release for a couple minutes, but then quick release.

When finished, check the temperature, making sure it's 165 degrees.

Remove chicken, and then shred it, and stir in the broth to flavor it, and then serve in bowls.

Nutritional information (per ½ cup): Calories: 169, Fat: 4g

Carbs: 5gNet Carbs: 1g Protein: 30g

Fiber: 3g Sodium 82%

Teriyaki Chicken

Preparation time: 8 minutes , Cook Time: 22 minutes

Serves: 4

Ingredients for Teriyaki sauce:

1/3 cup low-salt soy sauce

¼ cup honey

3 tablespoons arrowroot powder or corn starch

¼ cup rice wine vinegar or apple cider vinegar

¼ teaspoon dried sherry or mirin

3 tablespoons water for sauce

For chicken and rice:

1 tablespoon toasted sesame oil or olive oil

salt and black pepper for taste

½ teaspoon minced or grated ginger

1/3 cup shredded carrots

1 cup water

1/3 cup shelled edamame beans, thawed out

chopped green onions

1 medium boneless, skinless chicken breast

2 cloves minced garlic

¼ cup chopped red bell peppers

2 cups uncooked Jasmine rice washed, rinsed, and drained

1 cup broccoli florets

Sesame seeds to garnish

Directions:

Open instant pot and press sauté, and then whisk together the soy sauce, honey, vinegar, and mirin, and then, heat up the oil, and add the chicken, seasoning with salt and pepper, and sautéing for 2-3 minutes, until browned.

add ginger and garlic and cook for 20 seconds.

pour half the sauce into uncooked rice and one cup of water.

Cook on manual high pressure for 3 minutes, and then let it natural pressure release.

Add in the veggies and whisk the cornstarch slurry together and drizzle it over chicken

DASH DIET: THE COMPLETE GUIDE

and cook until veggies are tender, and sprinkle this with seeds and green onions, serving hot.

Nutrition facts: Calories: 419,

Fat: 6g Carbs: 81gNet Carbs: 79g

Protein: 8g Fiber: 2g Sodium 64%

Buffalo Chicken Quinoa bowls

Preparation time: 15 minutes , Cook Time: 15 minutes

Serves: 4

Ingredients:

3 pounds boneless, skinless chicken breasts

2 tablespoons olive oil

2 tablespoons hot sauce

2 tablespoons honey

4 tablespoons butter or ghee

1 cup buffalo wing sauce

4 cloves minced garlic

1 cup chopped green onions

For the Quinoa bowls

1 cup uncooked quinoa

1 sliced cucumber

2 chopped heads of lettuce

2.5 cups water

1 cup shredded carrots

1 sliced avocado

10 oz cherry tomatoes

Ranch dressing or another dressing to serve

Directions:

For the chicken, add the breasts, oil, butter or ghee, band everything else to the instant pot, cooking on manual high for 6 minutes.

Let it natural pressure release, and from there, let it cool for 5 minutes before you shred it carefully.

For the quinoa bowls, add the quinoa to the instant pot, and cook it for about 5 minutes, and then let it sit for 5 minutes then fluff.

Mix everything together, with the quinoa first, then the buffalo chicken, and then the rest.

Nutrition: Calories: 826 with fixings,

Fat: 30g Carbs: 60gNet Carbs: 48g

Protein: 72g Fiber: 12g Sodium 76%

Chicken Tacos

Preparation time: 5 minutes , Cook Time: 15 minutes

Servings: 4

Ingredients:

1 pound chicken breast

2 cloves garlic

2 cups fresh salsa

1 teaspoon meat

Directions:

Trim excess

Fat off chicken and put in instant pot.

Add salsa and garlic, and from there, turn on for 11 minutes poultry setting.

Release pressure naturally for 5 minutes, and from there, let it sit for 5 minutes before shredding.

Use fixings on top of this, or you can have naked tacos as needed.

Nutrition: Calories: 129, Fat: 3 g

Carbs: 4gNet Carbs: 3g Protein: 22g

Fiber: 1g Sodium 66%

Tuscan Chicken Pasta

Preparation time: 10 minutes , Cook Time: 4 minutes

Servings: 6

Ingredients:

3 cups low-Sodium chicken broth

½ tablespoon Italian seasoning

12 oz. Whole wheat noodles

1 cup cottage cheese

¼ teaspoon pepper

1/3 cup sun-dried tomatoes

1 tablespoon minced garlic

2 pounds chicken breast

2 cups spinach

1 cup plain Greek yogurt

¼ cup Parmesan

¼ cup basil

Directions:

Turn IP onto sauté and add the tomatoes, garlic, seasoning pepper, and salt, stirring for 30 seconds.

Add the chicken and brown for 1-2 minutes and keep the chicken from sticking.
add pasta and chicken broth and stir to cover it.

Manual cook it for 4 minutes, and then quick release the pressure, but be careful.

Blend the yogurt and cottage cheese and set it aside.

Stir pasta and noodles, and then add cheese, basil, and spinach, and mix it till everything is combined.

Pour cream over pasta, and then stir till all is covered.

Nutrition: Calories: 479,

Fat: 9g

Carbs: 49gNet

Carbs: 48g

Protein: 54g Fiber: 1g Sodium 52%

Pork Carnitas

Preparation time: 20 minutes , Cook Time: 80 minutes

Servings: 11

Ingredients:

3 pounds trimmed, boneless shoulder blade and roast, cut into pieces

salt and pepper for taste

6 cloves garlic, slivered

½ teaspoon sazon

2 teaspoons cumin

¼ teaspoon dried oregano

3 chipotle peppers in adobo sauce

¼ teaspoon dry adobo seasoning

1 cup reduced

Sodium chicken broth

2 bay leaves

½ teaspoon garlic powder

Directions:

Season pork with salt and pepper.

·Push sauté on instant pot, and then oil and brown the pork on every side, remove from heat to cool.

Using a knife, cut the roast about an inch deep and insert the slivers.

Season with everything else, and then add chipotle peppers, and then add bay leaves too.

Cook this in manual for 80 minutes, less time if the meat is smaller.

When finished, you shred the pork with two forks to combine it with juices.

Remove bay leaves and adjust cumin and add adobo sauce.

Nutrition: Calories: 160,

Fat: 7g

Carbs: 1gNet Carbs: 1g

Protein: 20g Fiber: 0g

Sodium 97%

Instant Pot Chipotle Burritos

Preparation time: 5 minutes, Cook Time: 30 minutes

Servings: 4

Ingredients:

1 cup dried black beans (don't soak them)

1 chipotle pepper from a can of adobo sauce

½ teaspoon dried oregano

sea salt

3 cups water

1 teaspoon cumin

1 cup brown rice

Lime and cilantro to garnish

Directions:

Add the beans, water, pepper, cumin, and oregano, and then in an oven-safe bowl, add the rice, salt, and about 1 ¼ cup of water, and put the trivet and rice on top of it.

From here, secure the lead, seal it, and manual cook it for 3-0 minutes, and from there, once finished, you should then vent it, and let it natural pressure release.

From there, remove everything and from there you can then mash the beans together with a masher, and you can further season them.

Serve this with your favorite burrito bowl toppings.

Nutrition: Calories: 339,

Fat: 2g

Carbs: 66gNet

Carbs: 54g

Protein: 15g

Fiber: 9g

Sodium 1%

Chapter 6 Dinner Recipes

Spinach Rolls

Preparation time: 10 minutes

Cooking time: 10 minutes

Servings: 4

Ingredients:

4 eggs, whisked

1/3 cup organic almond milk

½ teaspoon salt

½ teaspoon white pepper

1 teaspoon butter

9 oz chicken breast, boneless, skinless, cooked

2 cups spinach

2 tablespoon heavy cream

Directions:

Mix up together whisked eggs with almond milk and salt.

Preheat the skillet well and toss the butter in it.

Melt it.

Cook 4 crepes in the preheated skillet.

Meanwhile, chop the spinach and chicken breast.

Fill every egg crepe with chopped spinach, chicken breast, and heavy cream.

Roll the crepes and transfer on the serving plate.

Nutrition: calories 220,

Fat 14.5,

Fiber 0.8,

Carbs 2.4,

Protein 20.1

Sodium 31%

Goat Cheese Fold-Overs

Preparation time: 15 minutes

Cooking time: 8 minutes

Servings: 4

Ingredients:

8 oz goat cheese, crumbled

5 oz ham, sliced

1 cup almond flour

¼ cup of coconut milk

1 teaspoon olive oil

½ teaspoon dried dill

1 teaspoon Italian seasoning

½ teaspoon salt

Directions:

In the mixing bowl, mix up together almond flour, coconut milk, olive oil, and salt. You will get a smooth batter.

Preheat the non-stick skillet.

Separate batter into 4 parts. Pour 1st batter part in the preheated skillet and cook it for 1 minute from each side.

Repeat the same steps with all batter.

After this, mix up together crumbled goat cheese, dried dill, and Italian seasoning.

Spread every almond flour pancake with goat cheese mixture. Add sliced ham and fold them.

Nutrition: calories 402

Fat 31.8, Fiber 1.6, Carbs 5.1,

Protein 25.1   Sodium 69%

Crepe Pie

Preparation time: 10 minutes

Cooking time: 15 minutes

Servings: 8

Ingredients:

1 cup almond flour

1 cup coconut flour

½ cup heavy cream

1 teaspoon baking powder

½ teaspoon salt

10 oz ham, sliced

½ cup cream cheese

1 teaspoon chili flakes

1 tablespoon fresh cilantro, chopped

4 oz Cheddar cheese, shredded

Directions:

Make crepes: in the mixing bowl, mix up together almond flour, coconut flour, heavy cream, salt, and baking powder. Whisk the mixture.

Preheat the non-sticky skillet well and ladle 1 ladle of the crepe batter in it.

Make the crepes: cook them for 1 minute from each side over the medium heat.

Mix up together cream cheese, chili flakes, cilantro, and shredded Cheddar cheese.

After this, transfer 1st crepe in the plate. Spread it with cream cheese mixture. Add ham.

Repeat the steps until you use all the ingredients.

Bake the crepe pie for 5 minutes in the preheated to the 365F oven.

Cut it into the serving and serve hot.

Nutrition: calories 272,

Fat 18.8,

Fiber 6.9,

Carbs 13.2,

Protein 13.4

Sodium 59%

Coconut Soup

Preparation time: 15 minutes

Cooking time: 25 minutes

Servings: 4

Ingredients: 1 cup of coconut milk

2 cups of water 1 teaspoon curry paste

4 chicken thighs

½ teaspoon fresh ginger, grated

1 garlic clove, diced 1 teaspoon butter

1 teaspoon chili flakes

1 tablespoon lemon juice

Directions:

Toss the butter in the skillet and melt it.

Add diced garlic and grated ginger. Cook the ingredients for 1 minute. Stir them constantly.

Pour water in the saucepan. Add coconut milk and curry paste. Mix up the liquid until homogenous.

Add chicken thighs, chili flakes, and cooked ginger mixture. Close the lid and cook soup for 15 minutes.

Then start to whisk soup with the hand whisker and add lemon juice.

When all lemon juice is added, stop to whisk it. Close the lid and cook soup for 5 minutes more over the medium heat.

Then remove soup from the heat and let it rest for 15 minutes.

Nutrition: calories 318, Fat 26, Fiber 1.4, Carbs 4.2, Protein 20.6 Sodium 14%

Fish Tacos

Preparation time: 10 minutes

Cooking time: 5 minutes

Servings: 4

Ingredients:

4 lettuce leaves

½ red onion, diced

½ jalapeno pepper, minced

1 tablespoon olive oil

1-pound cod fillet

1 tablespoon lemon juice

¼ teaspoon ground coriander

Directions:

Sprinkle cod fillet with a ½ tablespoon of olive oil and ground coriander.

Preheat the grill well.

Grill the fish for 2 minutes from each side. The cooked fish has a light brown color.

After this, mix up together diced red onion, minced jalapeno pepper, remaining olive oil, and lemon juice.

Cut the grilled cod fillet into 4 pieces.

Place the fish in the lettuce leaves. Add mixed red onion mixture over the fish and transfer the tacos on the serving plates.

Nutrition: calories 157, Fat 4.5, Fiber 0.4,

Carbs 1.6, Protein 26.1 Sodium 37%

Sodium 43%

Cobb Salad

Preparation time: 10 minutes

Cooking time: 5 minutes

Servings: 2

Ingredients: 2 oz bacon, sliced

1 egg boiled, peeled

½ tomato, chopped

1 oz Blue cheese

1 teaspoon chives

1/3 cup lettuce, chopped

1 tablespoon mayonnaise

1 tablespoon lemon juice

Directions:

Place the bacon in the preheated skillet and roast it 1.5 minutes from each side.

When the bacon is cooked, chop it roughly and transfer in the salad bowl.

Chop the eggs roughly and add them in the salad bowl too.

After this, add chopped tomato, chives, and lettuce.

Chop Blue cheese and add it in the salad.

Then make seasoning: whisk together mayonnaise with lemon juice.

Pour the mixture over the salad and shake little.

Nutrition: calories 270, Fat 20.7,

Fiber 0.3, Carbs 3.7, Protein 16.6

Cheese Soup

Preparation time: 10 minutes

Cooking time:15 minutes

Servings: 3

Ingredients:

2 white onion, peeled, diced

1 cup Cheddar cheese, shredded

½ cup heavy cream

½ cup of water

1 teaspoon ground black pepper

1 tablespoon butter

½ teaspoon salt

Directions:

Pour water and heavy cream in the saucepan.

Bring it to boil.

Meanwhile, toss the butter in the pan, add diced onions and saute them.

When the onions are translucent, transfer them in the boiling liquid.

Add ground black pepper, salt, and cheese. Cook the soup for 5 minutes.

Then let it chill little and ladle it into the bowls.

Nutrition: calories 286,

Fat 23.8, Fiber 1.8, Carbs 8.3,

Protein 10.7 Sodium 29%

Tuna Tartare

Preparation time: 10 minutes

Servings: 4

Ingredients:

1-pound tuna steak

1 tablespoon mayonnaise

3 oz avocado, chopped

1 cucumber, chopped

1 tablespoon lemon juice

1 teaspoon cayenne pepper

1 teaspoon soy sauce

1 teaspoon chives

½ teaspoon cumin seeds

1 teaspoon canola oil

Directions:

Chop tuna steak and place it in the big bowl.

Add avocado, cucumber, and chives.

Mix up together lemon juice, cayenne pepper, soy sauce, cumin seeds, and canola oil.

Add mixed liquid in the tuna mixture and mix up well.

Place tuna tartare in the serving plates.

Nutrition: calories 292,

Fat 13.9, Fiber 2,

Carbs 6, Protein 35.1

Sodium 22%

Clam Chowder

Preparation time: 5 minutes

Cooking time: 15 minutes

Servings: 3

Ingredients: 1 cup of coconut milk

1 cup of water   6 oz clam, chopped

1 teaspoon chives   ½ teaspoon white pepper

¾ teaspoon chili flakes   ½ teaspoon salt

1 cup broccoli florets, chopped

Directions:

Pour coconut milk and water in the saucepan.

Add chopped clams, chives, white pepper, chili flakes, salt, and broccoli florets.

Close the lid and cook chowder over the medium-low heat for 15 minutes or until all the ingredients are soft.

It is recommended to serve the soup hot.

Nutrition: calories 139, Fat 9.8, Fiber 1.1,

Carbs 10.8, Protein 2.4   Sodium 44%

Asian Beef Salad

Preparation time: 10 minutes

Cooking time: 25 minutes

Servings: 4

Ingredients:

14 oz beef brisket

1 teaspoon sesame seeds

½ teaspoon cumin seeds

1 tablespoon apple cider vinegar

1 tablespoon avocado oil

1 red bell pepper, sliced

1 white onion, sliced

1 teaspoon butter

1 teaspoon ground black pepper

1 teaspoon soy sauce

1 garlic clove, sliced

1 cup water, for cooking

Directions:

Slice beef brisket and place it in the pan. Add water and close the lid.

Cook the beef for 25 minutes.

Then drain water and transfer beef brisket in the pan.

Add butter and roast it for 5 minutes.

Put the cooked beef brisket in the salad bowl.

Add sesame seeds, cumin seeds, apple cider vinegar, avocado oil, sliced bell pepper, onion, ground black pepper, and soy sauce.

Sprinkle the salad with garlic and mix it up.

Nutrition: calories 227,

Fat 8.1,

Fiber 1.4,

Carbs 6,

Protein 31.1

Sodium 83%

Carbonara

Preparation time: 10 minutes

Cooking time: 25 minutes

Servings: 6

Ingredients:

3 zucchini, trimmed

1 cup heavy cream

5 oz bacon, chopped

2 egg yolks

4 oz Cheddar cheese, grated

1 tablespoon butter

1 teaspoon chili flakes

1 teaspoon salt

½ cup water, for cooking

Directions:

Make the zucchini noodles with the help of the spiralizer.

Toss bacon in the skillet and roast it for 5 minutes on the medium heat. Stir it from time to time.

Meanwhile, in the saucepan, mix up together heavy cream, butter, salt, and chili flakes.

Add egg yolk and whisk the mixture until smooth.

Start to preheat the liquid, stir it constantly.

When the liquid starts to boil, add grated cheese and fried bacon. Mix it up and close the lid. Saute it on the low heat for 5 minutes.

Meanwhile, place the zucchini noodles in the skillet where bacon was and roast it for 3 minutes.

Then pour heavy cream mixture over zucchini and mix up well. Cook it for 1 minute more and transfer on the serving plates.

Nutrition: calories 324,

Fat 27.1,

Fiber 1.1,

Carbs 4.6,

Protein 16

Sodium 65%

Cauliflower Soup with Seeds

Preparation time: 10 minutes

Cooking time: 20 minutes

Servings: 4

Ingredients:

2 cups cauliflower

1 tablespoon pumpkin seeds

1 tablespoon chia seeds

½ teaspoon salt

1 teaspoon butter

¼ white onion, diced

½ cup coconut cream

1 cup of water

4 oz Parmesan, grated

1 teaspoon paprika

1 tablespoon dried cilantro

Directions:

Chop cauliflower and put in the saucepan.

Add salt, butter, diced onion, paprika, and dried cilantro.

Cook the cauliflower over the medium heat for 5 minutes.

Then add coconut cream and water.

Close the lid and boil soup for 15 minutes.

Then blend the soup with the help of hand blender.

Dring to boil it again.

Add grated cheese and mix up well.

Ladle the soup into the serving bowls and top every bowl with pumpkin seeds and chia seeds.

Nutrition: calories 214,

Fat 16.4,

Fiber 3.6, Carbs 8.1,

Protein 12.1 Sodium 43%

Prosciutto-Wrapped Asparagus

Preparation time: 15 minutes

Cooking time: 20 minutes

Servings: 6

Ingredients:

2-pound asparagus

8 oz prosciutto, sliced

1 tablespoon butter, melted

½ teaspoon ground black pepper

4 tablespoon heavy cream

1 tablespoon lemon juice

Directions:

Slice prousciutto slices into strips.

Wrap asparagus into prosciutto strips and place on the tray.

Sprinkle the vegetables with ground black pepper, heavy cream, and lemon juice. Add butter.

Preheat the oven to 365F.

Place the tray with asparagus in the oven and cook for 20 minutes.

Serve the cooked meal only hot.

Nutrition: calories 138,

Fat 7.9,

Fiber 3.2,

Carbs 6.9,

Protein 11.5

Sodium 3%

Stuffed Bell Peppers

Preparation time: 10 minutes

Cooking time: 25 minutes

Servings: 4

Ingredients: 4 bell peppers

1 ½ cup ground beef 1 zucchini, grated

1 white onion, diced

½ teaspoon ground nutmeg

1 tablespoon olive oil

1 teaspoon ground black pepper

½ teaspoon salt 3 oz Parmesan, grated

1.   Directions:

Cut the bell peppers into halves and remove seeds.

Place ground beef in the skillet.

Add grated zucchini, diced onion, ground nutmeg olive oil, ground black pepper, and salt.

Roast the mixture for 5 minutes.

Place bell pepper halves in the tray.

Fill every pepper half with ground beef mixture and top with grated Parmesan.

Cover the tray with foil and secure the edges.

Cook the stuffed bell peppers for 20 minutes at 360F.

Nutrition: calories 241,

Fat 14.6, Fiber 3.4,

Carbs 11, Protein 18.6 Sodium 37%

Stuffed Eggplants with Goat Cheese

Preparation time: 15 minutes

Cooking time: 25 minutes

Servings: 4

Ingredients:

1 large eggplant, trimmed

1 tomato, crushed

1 garlic clove, diced

½ teaspoon ground black pepper

½ teaspoon smoked paprika

1 cup spinach, chopped

4 oz goat cheese, crumbled

1 teaspoon butter

2 oz Cheddar cheese, shredded

Directions:

Cut the eggplants into halves and then cut every half into 2 parts.

Remove the flesh from the eggplants to get eggplant boards.

Mix up together crushed tomato, diced garlic, ground black pepper, smoked paprika, chopped spinach, crumbled goat cheese, and butter.

Fill the eggplants with this mixture.

Top every eggplant board with shredded Cheddar cheese.

Put the eggplants in the tray.

Preheat the oven to 365F.

Place the tray with eggplants in the oven and cook for 25 minutes.

Nutrition: calories 229,

Fat 16.1, Fiber 4.6,

Carbs 9, Protein 13.8 Sodium 21%

Korma Curry

Preparation time: 10 minutes

Cooking time: 25 minutes

Servings: 6

Ingredients:

3-pound chicken breast, skinless, boneless

1 teaspoon garam masala

1 teaspoon curry powder

1 tablespoon apple cider vinegar

½ coconut cream

1 cup organic almond milk

1 teaspoon ground coriander

¾ teaspoon ground cardamom

½ teaspoon ginger powder

¼ teaspoon cayenne pepper

¾ teaspoon ground cinnamon

1 tomato, diced 1 teaspoon avocado oil

½ cup of water

Directions:

Chop the chicken breast and put it in the saucepan.

Add avocado oil and start to cook it over the medium heat.

Sprinkle the chicken with garam masala, curry powder, apple cider vinegar, ground coriander, cardamom, ginger powder, cayenne pepper, ground cinnamon, and diced tomato. Mix up the ingredients carefully. Cook them for 10 minutes.

Add water, coconut cream, and almond milk. Saute the meal for 10 minutes more.

Nutrition: calories 411,

Fat 19.3,

Fiber 0.9,

Carbs 6,

Protein 49.9

Sodium 12%

Zucchini Bars

Preparation time: 10 minutes

Cooking time: 15 minutes

Servings: 8

Ingredients:

3 zucchini, grated

½ white onion, diced

2 teaspoons butter

3 eggs, whisked

4 tablespoons coconut flour

1 teaspoon salt

½ teaspoon ground black pepper

5 oz goat cheese, crumbled

4 oz Swiss cheese, shredded

½ cup spinach, chopped

1 teaspoon baking powder

½ teaspoon lemon juice

Directions:

In the mixing bowl, mix up together grated zucchini, diced onion, eggs, coconut flour, salt, ground black pepper, crumbled cheese, chopped spinach, baking powder, and lemon juice.

Add butter and churn the mixture until homogenous.

Line the baking dish with baking paper.

Transfer the zucchini mixture in the baking dish and flatten it.

Preheat the oven to 365F and put the dish inside.

Cook it for 15 minutes. Then chill the meal well.

Cut it into bars.

Nutrition: calories 199,

Fat 1316,

Fiber 215,

Carbs 7.1,

Protein 13.1

Sodium 21%

Mushroom Soup

Preparation time: 10 minutes

Cooking time: 25 minutes

Servings: 4

Ingredients: 1 cup of water

1 cup of coconut milk

1 cup white mushrooms, chopped

½ carrot, chopped

¼ white onion, diced

1 tablespoon butter

2 oz turnip, chopped

1 teaspoon dried dill

½ teaspoon ground black pepper

¾ teaspoon smoked paprika

1 oz celery stalk, chopped

Directions:

Pour water and coconut milk in the saucepan. Bring the liquid to boil. Add chopped mushrooms, carrot, and turnip. Close the lid and boil for 10 minutes. Meanwhile, put butter in the skillet. Add diced onion. Sprinkle it with dill, ground black pepper, and smoked paprika. Roast the onion for 3 minutes. Add the roasted onion in the soup mixture.

Then add chopped celery stalk. Close the lid.

Cook soup for 10 minutes.

Then ladle it into the serving bowls.

Nutrition: calories 181, Fat 17.3, Fiber 2.5,

Carbs 6.9, Protein 2.4 Sodium 4%

Stuffed Portobello Mushrooms

Preparation time: 10 minutes

Cooking time: 10 minutes

Servings: 4

Ingredients: 2 portobello mushrooms

1 cup spinach, chopped, steamed

2 oz artichoke hearts, drained, chopped

1 tablespoon coconut cream

1 tablespoon cream cheese

1 teaspoon minced garlic

1 tablespoon fresh cilantro, chopped

3 oz Cheddar cheese, grated

½ teaspoon ground black pepper

2 tablespoons olive oil

½ teaspoon salt

Directions:

Sprinkle mushrooms with olive oil and place in the tray. Transfer the tray in the preheated to 360F oven and broil them for 5 minutes. Meanwhile, blend together artichoke hearts, coconut cream, cream cheese, minced garlic, and chopped cilantro. Add grated cheese in the mixture and sprinkle with ground black pepper and salt. Fill the broiled mushrooms with the cheese mixture and cook them for 5 minutes more. Serve the mushrooms only hot.

Nutrition: calories 183, Fat 16.3, Fiber 1.9,

Carbs 3, Protein 7.7 Sodium 37%

Lettuce Salad

Preparation time: 10 minutes

Servings: 1

Ingredients:

1 cup Romaine lettuce, roughly chopped

3 oz seitan, chopped

1 tablespoon avocado oil

1 teaspoon sunflower seeds

1 teaspoon lemon juice

1 egg boiled, peeled

2 oz Cheddar cheese, shredded

Directions:

Place lettuce in the salad bowl. Add chopped seitan and shredded cheese.

Then chop the egg roughly and add in the salad bowl too.

Mix up together lemon juice with the avocado oil.

Sprinkle the salad with the oil mixture and sunflower seeds. Don't stir the salad before serving.

Nutrition: calories 663,

Fat 29.5,

Fiber 4.7,

Carbs 3.8,

Protein 84.2

Sodium 45%

Lemon Garlic Salmon

Preparation time: 3 minutes , Cook Time: 17 minutes

Servings: 4

Ingredients:

2 pounds salmon fillets, frozen

1 cup water

¼ teaspoon garlic powder

1/8 teaspoon pepper

1 tablespoon coconut oil

¼ cup lemon juice

sprigs of parsley

¼ teaspoon salt to taste

1 lemon

Directions:

Put water into IP and the lemon juice, then add the herbs, and put it in a steamer rack.

Drizzle salmon with oil and season with the pepper and salt.

Add garlic powder over salmon.

Layer the lemon slices over salmon.

Cook on manual high pressure for 7 minutes, then natural pressure release.

Enjoy over salad, or some roasted veggies!

Nutrition: Calories: 165,

Fat: 10gg Carbs: 8gNet Carbs: 4g

Protein: 15g Fiber: 4g Sodium 75%

Chickpea Curry

Preparation time: 10 minutes , Cook Time: 10 minutes

Servings: 6

Ingredients:

2 tablespoons olive oil

1 diced small green pepper

2 cans chickpeas, drained

1 cup corn,

1 cup kale leaves

1 tablespoon sugar-free maple syrup

1 diced onion

2 minced cloves of garlic

1 can diced tomatoes with juice

1 cup sliced okra

1 cup vegetable broth

1 teaspoon sea salt

Juice of a lime

¼ teaspoon ground black pepper

2 tablespoons cilantro leaves

Directions:

Turn on sauté function on IP.

Cook onion for four minutes till browned, and then add in garlic and pepper and cook for 2 more minutes.

Add in curry powder and stir for 30 seconds, and then add in rest of the ingredients, and seal the vent.

Manual pressure cook for 5 minutes, and then natural pressure release.

Add in the salt, pepper, and lime juice, and add more salt as needed.

Serve over cooked rice or top with cilantro leaves

Nutrition: Calories: 119,

Fat: 5g

Carbs: 18gNet

Carbs: 16g

Protein: 2g

Fiber: 2g

Sodium 30%

Instant Pot Chicken Thighs with Olives and Capers

Preparation time: 15 minutes, Cook Time: 20 minutes

Servings: 6

Ingredients:

6 chicken thighs

3 tablespoons avocado oil

¼ teaspoon sweet paprika

A couple small lemons

1 cup chicken stock

1 cup pitted olives

3 tablespoons parsley leaves for garnish

1 teaspoon kosher salt

1 teaspoon ground turmeric

¼ teaspoon black pepper

¼ teaspoon mustard powder

2 tablespoons cooking

Fat of choice

2 chopped cloves of garlic

2 tablespoons capers

Directions:

Season chicken thighs with salt and put them in baking dish.

Mix together the spices with the avocado oil and put it over the chicken and then put the marinate in there, and let it marinate for 20-30 minutes at room temperature.

Halve the lemons, and then heat the ghee, swirling to the pot bottom. Brown the chickens for 3 minutes undisturbed, and then brown the second side.

Do this with the rest of the chicken, and then use the broth to deglaze the pot.

Put lemons at the bottom and chicken over the top, and then the rest of the ingredients over chicken.

Let it cook for 14 minutes.

When finished, let natural pressure release, and then taste to see if it's ready, and put olives and capers over the chicken, garnishing with parsley.

Nutrition: Calories: 253,

Fat: 6g

Carbs: 10gNet

Carbs: 6g

Protein: 13g

Fiber: 4g

Sodium 60%

Instant Pot salmon

Preparation time: 5 minutes, Cook Time: 15 minutes

Servings: 4

Ingredients:

1 cup water

1 pound of salmon, cut into fillets

Salt and pepper to taste

Directions:

Put cup of water into the instant pot and add the trivet.

Put the fillets on top of that and add the salt and pepper onto it.

Secure and turn on the release valve to seal, and then cook manual high pressure for 3 minutes, or 5 minutes for frozen fillets.

When finished, let it vent and release the pressure, and serve with sauce or side dish.

Nutrition: Calories: 161,

Fat: 4g Carbs: 0, Net Carbs: 0,

Protein: 22g Fiber: 0g

Sodium 33%

Instant Pot Mac N' Cheese

Preparation time: 10 minutes, Cook Time: 10 minutes

Servings: 6

Ingredients:

1 cup raw cashews, soaked

¼ cup Nutritional yeast

1 tablespoon apple cider vinegar

12 ounces gluten-free pasta

5 cups water, divided

2 teaspoons sea salt

2 tablespoons lemon juice

1//4 teaspoon nutmeg

Directions:

Drain cashews and then combine cashews, 2 cups of water, yeast, lemon juice, vinegar, and nutmeg and then blend till smooth.

Add pasta to instant pot, and then put sauce on top, and then use two cups of water to rinse out the blender and then pour water from blender into instant pot, and then seal and cook on manual pressure for 0 minutes, then let it natural pressure release.

Release steam and then put rest of water into pot and use spoon to stir.

Adjust seasonings, and you can add veggies and such to this.

Nutrition: Calories: 329,

Fat: 10g Carbs: 52g Net Carbs: 50g

Protein: 7g Fiber: 2g Sodium 84%

Instant pot Mediterranean Chicken

Preparation time: 15 minutes , Cook Time: 5 minutes

Servings: 8

Ingredients:

8-10 organic, boneless and skinless chicken thighs

1 teaspoon paprika ¼ teaspoon chili powder

2 teaspoons dried parsley

Salt and pepper for taste

½ cup black olives 2 tablespoons olive oil

1 teaspoon onion powder

½ teaspoon coriander seed, ground

2 teaspoons dried oregano

1 can of dried and chopped tomatoes

Directions:

Set your IP to sauté, and then add the olive oil to the bottom to heat.Add chicken and sauté until it's browned, but not cooked.

Add onions and cook for 5 minutes, and then add all spices, tomatoes, and salt and pepper and cook for 3 minutes.

put the chicken back in and combine it together, manual cook for 8 minutes, and then let it naturally steam release, then put the black olives in to stir.

Can be served best over pasta, rice, veggies, or mashed potatoes and cauliflower.

Nutrition: Calories: 153, Fat: 8g Carbs: 9g Net Carbs: 7g Protein: 12g

Fiber: 2g Sodium 6%

Green Chicken and Rice Bowl

Preparation time: 10 minutes,

Cook Time: 32 minutes

Servings: 4

Ingredients:

1 cup chicken broth 3 cups water

½ teaspoon cumin, paprika, thyme, and turmeric

4 tablespoons hummus

½ cup Kalamata olives

2 chicken breasts, skinless

2 cups basmati rice

½ teaspoon red pepper

salt and pepper for taste

4 tablespoons tzatziki sauce

4 tablespoons feta cheese

Directions:

Season chicken with spices.

Add chicken to instant pot with the broth.

Cook on manual high pressure, then release naturally for 10 minutes. Remove chicken and then shred chicken. Rinse rice and then add it to instant pot, cooking for 22 minutes on high pressure, then natural pressure release. Add the rice, chicken, and the rest of the ingredients to make rice bowl.

Nutrition: Calories: 426, Fat: 10g

Carbs: 12gNet Carbs: 5g Protein: 25g

Fiber: 7g Sodium 59%

Turkey Meatballs with Spaghetti Squash

Preparation time: 15 minutes, Cook Time: 25 minutes

Servings: 6

Ingredients:

1 pound ground chicken or turkey

5 cloves grated garlic

3 ounces diced prosciutto,

½ teaspoon dried cumin

2 slices whole grain bread

An egg

½ cup ricotta cheese

1 teaspoon dried oregano

½ teaspoon red pepper flakes

2 tablespoons extra virgin olive oil

¼ cup red wine

1 Parmesan rind

A pinch of kosher salt and pepper

2 cans crushed tomatoes

1 small spaghetti squash

2 sprigs thyme

Directions:

Preheat broiler to high and line with parchment paper.

Add the ground turkey and then run bread over till dampened, and then squeeze out excess water, and crumble bread over turkey.

Add rest of the ingredients and create small balls with hands.

Broil this for 3-4 minutes till browned.

In instant pot, put the garlic, tomatoes, water, and a pinch of salt and pepper, and then put the spaghetti squash in there, and from there, add meatballs.

Add the rest and cook on high pressure for 30 minutes, and then natural pressure release.

Remove squash and cut it till it's in half, and then scrape squash into strands, and then divide it into plates and top with basil and parmesan.

Nutrition: Calories: 326, Fat: 5g

Carbs: 20gNet Carbs: 16g Protein: 15g

Fiber: 4g Sodium 37%

Instant Pot Chicken Parmesan

Preparation time: 5 minutes , Cook Time: 15 minutes

Servings: 4

Ingredients:

1 pound chicken, cubed

1 medium jar marinara sauce

½ teaspoon Italian seasoning

¼ teaspoon basil

½ teaspoon garlic powder

salt and pepper for taste

½ cup mozzarella cheese

Directions:

turn on sauté on instant pot till hot, and then add 2 tablespoons olive oil, and then chicken and sauté for about 3-5 minutes.

Hit cancel and then cook the chicken in some marinara sauce for 5 minutes on high pressure, then natural pressure release.

You can from there serve this over some zoodles with mozzarella cheese, but let it rest in keep warm.

You can also use this on baked sandwiches and then cook it for 10 minutes.

Nutrition: Calories: 175,

Fat: 6g Carbs: 3gNet Carbs: 1g

Protein: 10g Fiber: 2g Sodium 14%

Instant Pot Chicken Marsala

Preparation time 15 minutes, Cook Time: 30 minutes

Servings: 5

Ingredients:

¼ cup flour

1 tsp garlic powder

2 pounds boneless, skinless chicken breasts, pounded

8 oz. Portobello mushrooms

¾ cup marsala wine

¼ cup heavy cream

2 teaspoons Italian seasoning

salt and pepper for taste

3 tablespoons extra virgin olive oil

2 tablespoons butter

½ chopped red onion

1 cup chicken broth

1.4 cup chopped parsley

4 oz. Room temp cream cheese

Directions:

Put the flour, seasoning and powder in a bowl, seasoning with salt and pepper.

Put chicken in there and seal it and move it around till coated.

Press sauté, and then set to high, adding the oil, and then add chicken to bottom, and brown them 3 minutes a side.

Once butter is put in, add the mushrooms and onion, stirring until they are browned and softened.

Add the marsala wine and chicken broth to deglaze bottom.

Turn IP off and add brown chicken to side, and from there, set it to pot once cleaned. Cook on manual high for 10 minutes.

Once finished, let it release naturally for 10 minutes, then quick for five, let chicken cool for 5 minutes.

Top every chicken with mushroom.

Nutrition: Calories: 270,

Fat: 5g Carbs: 3gNet

Carbs: 3g Protein: 15g

Fiber: 0g   Sodium 55%

Instant Pot Sausage Chicken Casserole

Preparation time 30 minutes, Cook Time: 30 minutes

Servings: 6

Ingredients:

2 celery stalks

2 cloves garlic

3 tablespoons butter

8 oz. Cream cheese

1 cup cheddar and Colby jack cheese, shredded

½ yellow onion

1 head of cauliflower

1 pound breakfast sausage

1 pound shredded chicken

1 teaspoon salt

½ teaspoon ground pepper

½ teaspoon paprika

1 cup water

Directions:

Chop your veggies and pre-heat oven to sauté.

Add butter, and sauté the onion, celery, and garlic for 305 minutes, then add the sausage in, and the cream cheese, and shredded chicken, finally the rest of the ingredients to instant pot, with a cup of water.

Turn off sauté, then go manual, 8 minutes natural pressure release. From there, stir it together, and if there is water, turn on sauté to further cook it a little.

Top with basil and parsley and enjoy!

Nutrition: Calories 683, Fat 57g Carbs9gNet

Carbs 7g Protein 32g Fiber 2g

Sodium 90%

Spicy Pasta

Preparation time: 10 minutes, Cook Time: 20 minutes

Serves: 4

Ingredients:

¼ cup divided olive oil

3 cloves minced garlic

1 can crushed tomatoes

2 tablespoons minced parsley

1 cup grated Romano cheese

1 medium head of cauliflower, trimmed

1 large sliced yellow onion

1 teaspoon crushed red pepper

1 pound whole-wheat pasta

Directions:

Take the oil ad add the cauliflower and garlic, sautéing until browned.

Add the rest of the olive oil and the sliced onion and cook it until browned as well.

Add the tomatoes and pepper to the mixture and cook till it starts to thicken.

Add in the pasta, and cook on manual mode for 5 minutes, natural pressure release. You may need more water depending on size.

When finished, mix it together and then stir in parsley and cheese.

Nutrition: Calories 138,

Fat 6g

Carbs 12gNet

Carbs 10g

Protein 4g

Fiber 4g

Sodium 19%

Chapter 7 Dessert Recipes

Hearty Cashew and Almond butter

Servings: 1 and ½ cups

Preparation Time: 5 minutes

Cooking Time: Nil

Ingredients:

1 cup almonds, blanched

1/3 cup cashew nuts

2 tablespoons coconut oil

Sunflower seeds as needed

½ teaspoon cinnamon

Directions:

Pre-heat your oven to 350 degrees F.

Bake almonds and cashews for 12 minutes.

Let them cool.

Transfer to food processor and add remaining ingredients.

Add oil and keep blending until smooth.

Serve and enjoy!

Nutrition:

Calories: 205

Fat: 19g Carbohydrates: g Protein: 2.8g

Sodium 9%

The Refreshing Nutter

Servings: 1

Preparation Time: 10 minutes

Ingredients:

1 tablespoon chia seeds

2 cups water

1 ounces Macadamia Nuts

1-2 packets Stevia, optional

1 ounce hazelnut

Directions:

Add all the listed ingredients to a blender.

Blend on high until smooth and creamy.

Enjoy your smoothie.

Nutrition:

Calories: 452

Fat: 43g

Carbohydrates: 15g

Protein: 9g

Sodium 1%

Elegant Cranberry Muffins

Servings: 24muffins

Preparation Time: 10 minutes

Cooking Time: 20 minutes

Ingredients:

2 cups almond flour

2 teaspoons baking soda ¼ cup avocado oil

1 whole egg ¾ cup almond milk

½ cup Erythritol   ½ cup apple sauce

Zest of 1 orange

2 teaspoons ground cinnamon

2 cup fresh cranberries

Directions:

Pre-heat your oven to 350 degrees F.

Line muffin tin with paper muffin cups and keep them on the side.

Add flour, baking soda and keep it on the side.

Take another bowl and whisk in remaining ingredients and add flour, mix well.

Pour batter into prepared muffin tin and bake for 20 minutes.

Once done, let it cool for 10 minutes.

Serve and enjoy!

Nutrition: Total Carbs: 7g   Fiber: 2g

Protein: 2.3g   Fat: 7g

Sodium 77%

Apple and Almond Muffins

Servings: 6 muffins

Preparation Time: 10 minutes

Cooking Time: 20 minutes

Ingredients:

6 ounces ground almonds

1 teaspoon cinnamon

½ teaspoon baking powder

1 pinch sunflower seeds

1 whole egg

1 teaspoon apple cider vinegar

2 tablespoons Erythritol

1/3 cup apple sauce

Directions:

Pre-heat your oven to 350 degrees F.

Line muffin tin with paper muffin cups, keep them on the side.

Mix in almonds, cinnamon, baking powder, sunflower seeds and keep it on the side.

Take another bowl and beat in eggs, apple cider vinegar, apple sauce, Erythritol.

Add the mix to dry ingredients and mix well until you have a smooth batter.

Pour batter into tin and bake for 20 minutes.

Once done, let them cool.

Serve and enjoy!

Nutrition: Total Carbs: 10   Fiber: 4g

Protein: 13g   Fat: 17g Sodium 47%

Stylish Chocolate Parfait

Servings: 4

Preparation Time: 2 hours

Cooking Time: nil

Ingredients:

2 tablespoons cocoa powder

1 cup almond milk

1 tablespoon chia seeds

Pinch of sunflower seeds

½ teaspoon vanilla extract

Directions:

Take a bowl and add cocoa powder, almond milk, chia seeds, vanilla extract and stir.

Transfer to dessert glass and place in your fridge for 2 hours.

Serve and enjoy!

Nutrition:

Calories: 130

Fat: 5g

Carbohydrates: 7g

Protein: 16g

Sodium 4%

Supreme Matcha Bomb

Servings: 10

Preparation Time: 100 minutes

Cooking Time: Nil

Ingredients:

3/4 cup hemp seeds

½ cup coconut oil

2 tablespoons coconut almond butter

1 teaspoon Matcha powder

2 tablespoons vanilla bean extract

½ teaspoon mint extract

Liquid stevia

Directions:

Take your blender/food processor and add hemp seeds, coconut oil, Matcha, vanilla extract and stevia.

Blend until you have a nice batter and divide into silicon molds.

Melt coconut almond butter and drizzle on top.

Let the cups chill and enjoy!

Nutrition:

Calories: 200

Fat: 20g

Carbohydrates: 3g

Protein: 5g

Sodium 6%

Mesmerizing Avocado and Chocolate Pudding

Servings: 2

Preparation Time: 30 minutes

Cooking Time: Nil

Ingredients:

1 avocado, chunked

1 tablespoon natural sweetener such as stevia

2 ounces cream cheese, at room temp

¼ teaspoon vanilla extract

4 tablespoons cocoa powder, unsweetened

Directions:

Blend listed ingredients in blender until smooth.

Divide the mix between dessert bowls, chill for 30 minutes.

Serve and enjoy!

Nutrition: Calories: 281 Fat: 27g

Carbohydrates: 12g Protein: 8g

Sodium 18%

Hearty Pineapple Pudding

Servings: 4

Preparation Time: 10 minutes

Cooking Time: 5 hours

Ingredients:

1 teaspoon baking powder

1 cup coconut flour

3 tablespoons stevia

3 tablespoons avocado oil

½ cup coconut milk

½ cup pecans, chopped

½ cup pineapple, chopped

½ cup lemon zest, grated

1 cup pineapple juice, natural

Directions:

Grease Slow Cooker with oil.

Take a bowl and mix in flour, stevia, baking powder, oil, milk, pecans, pineapple, lemon zest, pineapple juice and stir well.

Pour the mix into the Slow Cooker.

Place lid and cook on LOW for 5 hours.

Divide between bowls and serve.

Enjoy!

Nutrition:

Calories: 188

Fat: 3g

Carbohydrates: 14g

Protein: 5g

Sodium 5%

Healthy Berry Cobbler

Servings: 8

Preparation Time: 10 minutes

Cooking Time: 2 hours 30 minutes

Ingredients:

1 ¼ cups almond flour

1 cup coconut sugar

1 teaspoon baking powder

½ teaspoon cinnamon powder

1 whole egg

¼ cup low-

Fat milk

2 tablespoons olive oil

2 cups raspberries

2 cups blueberries

Directions:

Take a bowl and add almond flour, coconut sugar, baking powder and cinnamon.

Stir well .

Take another bowl and add egg milk, oil, raspberries, blueberries and stir.

Combine both of the mixtures.

Grease your Slow Cooker.

Pour the combined mixture into your Slow Cooker and cook on HIGH for 2 hours 30 minutes.

Divide between serving bowls and enjoy!

Nutrition: Calories: 250 Fat: 4g

Carbohydrates: 30g Protein: 3g

Sodium 1%

Tasty Poached Apples

Servings: 8

Preparation Time: 10 minutes

Cooking Time: 2 hours 30 minutes

Ingredients:

6 apples, cored, peeled and sliced

1 cup apple juice, natural

1 cup coconut sugar

1 tablespoon cinnamon powder

Directions:

Grease Slow Cooker with cooking spray.

Add apples, sugar, juice, cinnamon to your Slow Cooker.

Stir gently.

Place lid and cook on HIGH for 4 hours.

Serve cold and enjoy!

Nutrition: Calories: 180 Fat: 5g

Carbohydrates: 8g Protein: 4g

Sodium 2%

Home Made Trail Mix For The Trip

Servings: 4

Preparation Time: 10 minutes

Cooking Time: 55 minutes

Ingredients: ¼ cup raw cashews

¼ cup almonds ¼ cup walnuts

1 teaspoon cinnamon

2 tablespoons melted coconut oil

Sunflower seeds as needed

Directions:

Line baking sheet with parchment paper. Pre-heat your oven to 275 degrees F. Melt coconut oil and keep it on the side. Combine nuts to large mixing bowl and add cinnamon and melted coconut oil. Stir. Sprinkle sunflower seeds. Place in oven and brown for 6 minutes. Enjoy!

Nutrition: Calories: 363   Fat: 22g Carbohydrates: 41g   Protein: 7g   Sodium 13%

Heart Warming Cinnamon Rice Pudding

Servings: 4

Preparation Time: 10 minutes

Cooking Time: 5 hours

Ingredients: 6 ½ cups water

1 cup coconut sugar 2 cups white rice

2 cinnamon sticks ½ cup coconut, shredded

Directions:

Add water, rice, sugar, cinnamon and coconut to your Slow Cooker. Gently stir. Place lid and cook on HIGH for 5 hours. Discard cinnamon. Divide pudding between dessert dishes and enjoy!

Nutrition: Calories: 173

Fat: 4g Carbohydrates: 9g

Protein: 4g Sodium 12%

Pure Avocado Pudding

Servings: 4

Preparation Time: 3 hours

Cooking Time: nil

Ingredients: 1 cup almond milk

2 avocados, peeled and pitted

¾ cup cocoa powder

1 teaspoon vanilla extract

2 tablespoons stevia ¼ teaspoon cinnamon

Walnuts, chopped for serving

Directions:

Add avocados to a blender and pulse well.

Add cocoa powder, almond milk, stevia, vanilla bean extract and pulse the mixture well. Pour into serving bowls and top with walnuts. Chill for 2-3 hours and serve!

Nutrition: Calories: 221 Fat: 8g

Carbohydrates: 7g Protein: 3g

Sodium 10%

Sweet Almond and Coconut Fat Bombs

Servings: 6

Preparation Time: 10 minutes

Cooking Time: 0 mins

Freeze Time: 20 minutes

Ingredients: ¼ cup melted coconut oil

9 ½ tablespoons almond butter

90 drops liquid stevia

3 tablespoons cocoa

9 tablespoons melted almond butter, sunflower seeds

Directions: Take a bowl and add all of the listed ingredients. Mix them well.

Pour 2 tablespoons of the mixture into as many muffin molds as you like.

Chill for 20 minutes and pop them out. Serve and enjoy!

Nutrition: Total Carbs: 2g Fiber: 0g

Protein: 2.53g Fat: 14g

Sodium 78%

Spicy Popper Mug Cake

Servings: 2

Preparation Time: 5 minutes

Cooking Time: 5 minutes

Ingredients:

2 tablespoons almond flour

1 tablespoon flaxseed meal

1 tablespoon almond butter

1 tablespoon cream cheese

1 large egg

1 bacon, cooked and sliced

½ jalapeno pepper

½ teaspoon baking powder

¼ teaspoon sunflower seeds

Directions:

Take a frying pan and place it over medium heat.

Add slice of bacon and cook until it has a crispy texture.

Take a microwave proof container and mix all of the listed ingredients (including cooked bacon), clean the sides.

Microwave for 75 seconds, making to put your microwave to high power.

Take out the cup and tap it against a surface to take the cake out.

Garnish with a bit of jalapeno and serve!

Nutrition:

Calories: 429

Fat: 38g

Carbohydrates: 6g

Protein: 16g

Sodium 20%

The Most Elegant Parsley Soufflé Ever

Servings: 5

Preparation Time: 5 minutes

Cooking Time: 6 minutes

Ingredients:

2 whole eggs

1 fresh red chili pepper, chopped

2 tablespoons coconut cream

1 tablespoon fresh parsley, chopped

Sunflower seeds to taste

Directions:

Pre-heat your oven to 390 degrees F.

Almond butter 2 soufflé dishes.

Add the ingredients to a blender and mix well.

Divide batter into soufflé dishes and bake for 6 minutes.

Serve and enjoy!

Nutrition:

Calories: 108

Fat: 9g

Carbohydrates: 9g

Protein: 6g

Sodium 14%

Fennel and Almond Bites

Servings: 12

Preparation Time: 10 minutes

Cooking Time: None

Freeze Time:3 hours

Ingredients:

1 teaspoon vanilla extract

¼ cup almond milk

¼cup cocoa powder

½ cup almond oil

A pinch of sunflower seeds

1 teaspoon fennel seeds

Directions:

Take a bowl and mix the almond oil and almond milk.

Beat until smooth and glossy using electric beater.

Mix in the rest of the ingredients.

Take a piping bag and pour into a parchment paper lined baking sheet.

Freeze for 3 hours and store in the fridge.

Nutrition:

Total

Carbs: 1g

Fiber: 1g

Protein: 1g

Fat: 20g Sodium 3%

Feisty Coconut Fudge

Servings: 12

Preparation Time: 20 minutes

Cooking Time: None

Freeze Time: 2 hours

Ingredients:

¼ cup coconut, shredded

2 cups coconut oil

½ cup coconut cream

¼ cup almonds, chopped

1 teaspoon almond extract

A pinch of sunflower seeds

Stevia to taste

Directions:

Take a large bowl and pour coconut cream and coconut oil into it.

Whisk using an electric beater.

Whisk until the mixture becomes smooth and glossy.

Add cocoa powder slowly and mix well.

Add in the rest of the ingredients.

Pour into a bread pan lined with parchment paper.

Freeze until set.

Cut them into squares and serve.

Nutrition:

Total Carbs: 1g Fiber: 1g Protein: 0g

Fat: 20g Sodium 5%

No Bake Cheesecake

Servings: 10

Preparation Time: 120 minutes

Cooking Time: Nil

Ingredients: For Crust

2 tablespoons ground flaxseeds

2 tablespoons desiccated coconut

1 teaspoon cinnamon

For Filling

4 ounces vegan cream cheese

1 cup cashews, soaked

½ cup frozen blueberries

2 tablespoons coconut oil

1 tablespoon lemon juice

1 teaspoon vanilla extract

Liquid stevia

Directions:

Take a container and mix in the crust ingredients, mix well.

Flatten the mixture at the bottom to prepare the crust of your cheesecake.

Take a blender/ food processor and add the filling ingredients, blend until smooth.

Gently pour the batter on top of your crust and chill for 2 hours. Serve and enjoy!

Nutrition:

Calories: 182 Fat: 16g Carbohydrates: 4g

Protein: 3g Sodium 36%

Easy Chia Seed Pumpkin Pudding

Servings: 4

Preparation Time: 10-15 minutes/ overnight chill time

Cooking Time: Nil

Ingredients:

1 cup maple syrup

2 teaspoons pumpkin spice

1 cup pumpkin puree

1 ¼ cup almond milk

½ cup chia seeds

Directions:

Add all of the ingredients to a bowl and gently stir.

Let it refrigerate overnight or at least 15 minutes.

Top with your desired ingredients, such as blueberries, almonds, etc.

Serve and enjoy!

Nutrition:

Calories: 230

Fat: 10g

Carbohydrates:22g

Protein:11g

Sodium 37%

4 tablespoons fresh lime juice

10 tablespoons water

Directions:

Add all of the listed ingredients to a blender (except blueberries) and pulse the mixture well.

Transfer the mix into small serving bowls and chill the bowls.

Serve with a topping of blueberries.

Enjoy!

Nutrition:

Calories: 166

Fat: 13g

Carbohydrates: 13g

Protein: 1.7g

Sodium 2%

Lovely Blueberry Pudding

Servings: 4

Preparation Time: 20 minutes

Cooking Time: Nil

Smart Points: 0

Ingredients:

2 cups frozen blueberries

2 teaspoons lime zest, grated freshly

20 drops liquid stevia

2 small avocados, peeled, pitted and chopped

½ teaspoon fresh ginger, grated freshly

Decisive Lime and Strawberry Popsicle

Servings: 4

Preparation Time: 2 hours

Cooking Time: Nil

Ingredients:

1 tablespoon lime juice, fresh

¼ cup strawberries, hulled and sliced

¼ cup coconut almond milk, unsweetened and full

Fat

2 teaspoons natural sweetener

Directions:

Blend the listed ingredients in a blender until smooth.

Pour mix into popsicle molds and let them chill for 2 hours.

Serve and enjoy!

Nutrition:

Calories: 166

Fat: 17g

Carbohydrates: 3g

Protein: 1g

Sodium 2%

Ravaging Blueberry Muffin

Servings: 4

Preparation Time: 10 minutes

Cooking Time: 30 minutes

Ingredients:

1 cup almond flour

Pinch of sunflower seeds

1/8 teaspoon baking soda

1 whole egg

2 tablespoons coconut oil, melted

½ cup coconut almond milk

¼ cup fresh blueberries

Directions:

Pre-heat your oven to 350 degrees F.

Line a muffin tin with paper muffin cups.

Add almond flour, sunflower seeds, baking soda to a bowl and mix, keep it on the side.

Take another bowl and add egg coconut oil, coconut almond milk and mix.

Add mix to flour mix and gently combine until incorporated.

Mix in blueberries and fill the cupcakes tins with batter.

Bake for 20-25 minutes.

Enjoy!

Nutrition:

Calories: 167   Fat: 15g Carbohydrates: 2.1g Protein: 5.2g Sodium 13%

The Coconut Loaf

Servings: 4

Preparation Time: 15 minutes

Cooking Time: 40 minutes

Ingredients:

1 ½ tablespoons coconut flour

¼ teaspoon baking powder

1/8 teaspoon sunflower seeds

1 tablespoons coconut oil, melted

1 whole egg

Directions:

Pre-heat your oven to 350 degrees F.

Add coconut flour, baking powder, sunflower seeds.

Add coconut oil, eggs and stir well until mixed.

Leave batter for several minutes.

Pour half batter onto baking pan.

Spread it to form a circle, repeat with remaining batter.

Bake in oven for 10 minutes.

Once you have a golden brown texture, let it cool and serve.

Enjoy!

Nutrition:

Calories: 297 Fat: 14g

Carbohydrates: 15g Protein: 15g

Sodium 8%

Fresh Figs with Walnuts and Ricotta

Servings: 4

Preparation Time: 5 minutes

Cooking Time: 2-3 minutes

Ingredients:

8 dried figs, halved

¼ cup ricotta cheese

16 walnuts, halved

1 tablespoon honey

Directions:

Take a skillet and place it over medium heat, add walnuts and toast for 2 minutes.

Top figs with cheese and walnuts.

Drizzle honey on top.

Enjoy!

Nutrition:

Calories: 142

Fat: 8g

Carbohydrates:10g

Protein:4g

Sodium 5%

Authentic Medjool Date Truffles

Servings: 4

Preparation Time: 10-15 minutes

Cooking Time: Nil

Ingredients:

2 tablespoons peanut oil

½ cup popcorn kernels

1/3 cup peanuts, chopped

1/3 cup peanut almond butter

¼ cup wildflower honey

Directions:

Take a pot and add popcorn kernels, peanut oil.

Place it over medium heat and shake the pot gently until all corn has popped.

Take a saucepan and add honey, gently simmer for 2-3 minutes.

Add peanut almond butter and stir.

Coat popcorn with the mixture and enjoy!

Nutrition:

Calories: 430

Fat: 20g

Carbohydrates: 56g

Protein 9g

Sodium 69%

Tasty Mediterranean Peanut Almond butter Popcorns

Servings: 4

Preparation Time: 5 minutes + 20 minutes chill time

Cooking Time: 2-3 minutes

Ingredients:

3 cups Medjool dates, chopped

12 ounces brewed coffee

1 cup pecans, chopped

½ cup coconut, shredded

½ cup cocoa powder

Directions:

Soak dates in warm coffee for 5 minutes.

Remove dates from coffee and mash them, making a fine smooth mixture.

Stir in remaining ingredients (except cocoa powder) and form small balls out of the mixture.

Coat with cocoa powder, serve and enjoy!

Nutrition:

Calories: 265

Fat: 12g

Carbohydrates: 43g

Protein 3g

Sodium 9%

Just A Minute Worth Muffin

Servings: 2

Preparation Time: 5 minutes

Cooking Time: 1 minute

Ingredients:

Coconut oil for grease

2 teaspoons coconut flour

1 pinch baking soda

1 pinch sunflower seeds

1 whole egg

Directions:

Grease ramekin dish with coconut oil and keep it on the side.

Add ingredients to a bowl and combine until no lumps.

Pour batter into ramekin.

Microwave for 1 minute on HIGH.

Slice in half and serve.

Enjoy!

Nutrition:

Total

Carbs: 5.4

Fiber: 2g

Protein: 7.3g

Sodium 8%

Hearty Almond Bread

Servings: 8

Preparation Time: 15 minutes

Cooking Time: 60 minutes

Ingredients:

3 cups almond flour

1 teaspoon baking soda

2 teaspoons baking powder

¼ teaspoon sunflower seeds

¼ cup almond milk

½ cup + 2 tablespoons olive oil

3 whole eggs

Directions:

Pre-heat your oven to 300 degrees F.

Take a 9x5 inch loaf pan and grease, keep it on the side.

Add listed ingredients to a bowl and pour the batter into the loaf pan.

Bake for 60 minutes.

Once baked, remove from oven and let it cool.

Slice and serve!

Nutrition:

Calories: 277

Fat: 21g

Carbohydrates: 7g

Protein: 10g

Sodium 23%

Lemon Granita

Servings: 10

Preparation Time: 10 minutes

Ingredients

4 fresh lemons, juice about 3/4 cup

1 ½ cups of natural sweetener (Stevia, Erythritol...etc.)

3 cups water

2 lemon peeled, pulp

Directions:

In a saucepan, heat all Ingredients over medium heat.

Remove from heat and let cool on room temperature.

Pour the mixture in a baking dish, wrap with plastic membrane and freeze for 6 - 8 hours.

Remove granita from the freezer, scratch with big fork and stir.

Serve in chilled glasses and enjoy!

Keep in freezer.

Nutrition:

Calories: 13

Carbohydrates: 3g

Proteins: 1g

Fat: 1g

Fiber: 0.2g

Sodium 3%

Low Carb Blackberry Ice Cream

Servings: 8

Preparation Time: 10 minutes

Ingredients

3/4 lbs. of frozen blackberries, unsweetened

1 1/4 cup of caned coconut milk

1/4 cup of granulated Stevia sweetener or to taste

2 Tbsp of almond flour

1 pinch of ground vanilla

1 Tbsp of MCT oil

Directions:

Put all the Ingredients in a blender. Make sure blackberries are still frozen.

Blend until the mixture is creamy.

Pour the blackberry mixture in a container and freeze overnight.

Serve in chilled glasses or bowls.

Nutrition:

Calories: 83

Carbohydrates: 5g

Proteins: 1g

Fat: 8g

Fiber: 2.5g

Sodium 10%

Chocolate Coconut Ice Cream

Servings: 8

Preparation Time: 15 minutes

Ingredients

2 can (11 oz) of frozen coconut milk

2 scoop powdered chocolate

Protein

4 Tbsp of stevia sweetener

2 Tbsp of cocoa powder

Directions:

In a high-speed blender, stir the iced coconut milk.

Blend for 30 - 45 seconds and then add the remaining Ingredients.

Blend again until get a thick cream.

Pour the mixture in a container and store in freezer for 4 hours.

To prevent forming ice crystals, beat the mixture every 30 minutes.

Ready! Serve in chilled glasses.

Nutrition:

Calories: 135

Carbohydrates: 3g

Proteins: 4g

Fat: 15g

Fiber: 1g

Sodium 6%

Chocolate Peppermint Popsicles

Servings: 8

Preparation Time: 20 minutes

Ingredients 2 gelatin sheets

3 cups coconut milk (canned), divided

3 cup packed peppermint leaves

1 cup stevia granulate sweetener

1/4 tsp pure peppermint extract

3/4 cup of dark chocolate (60- 69% of cacao solid) melted

Directions:

Soak gelatin in a little coconut milk for 10 minutes.

In a saucepan, heat the coconut milk and peppermint leaves; cook for 3 minutes stirring constantly. Add soaked gelatin and stir until completely dissolved. Remove the saucepan from heat, cover and set aside for 20 - 25 minutes. Strain the mint mixture through a colander into the bowl and add the stevia sweetener: stir well. Pour the peppermint extract and stir.

Place bowl in the freezer for about one hour.

Remove from freezer and stir melted dark chocolate. Pour into Popsicle molds, insert sticks in each mold, and freeze overnight.

Remove popsicles from the mold and serve.

Nutrition:

Calories: 231 Carbohydrates: 8g Proteins: 3g

Fat: 22g Fiber: 1g Sodium 42%

Perfect Strawberry Ice Cream

Servings: 12

Preparation Time: 20 minutes

Ingredients

2 lbs. of strawberries

2 1/4 cups of water

2 Tbsp of coconut butter, softened

1 1/2 cups of natural granulated sweetener (Stevia, Truvia, Erythritol...etc.)

2 egg whites

Juice of 1 large lemon

Directions:

Heat strawberries, water, coconut butter and stevia sweetener in a saucepan over medium-low heat.

When strawberries softened, remove the saucepan from heat, and allow it to cool on room temperature.

Whisk the egg whites until stiff; add the lemon juice and stir. Add the egg whites mixture to strawberry mixture and gently stir with wooden spatula.

Refrigerate the ice cream mixture for 2 hours. Pour cold ice cream mixture into ice cream maker, turn on the machine, and do according to manufacturer's directions.

In the case that you do not have ice cream maker, pour the mixture in a container and freeze for 8 hours.

Nutrition:

Calories: 50 Carbohydrates: 6g Proteins: 1g

Fat: 5g Fiber: 2g Sodium 21%

Raskolnikov Vanilla Ice Cream

Servings: 8

Preparation Time: 10 minutes

Cooking Time: 20 minutes

Ingredients 3 sheets of gelatin sugar-free

2 US pints of cream 1/2 vanilla stick

1/2 cup stevia granulated sweetener

4 egg yolks 3 Tbsp of vodka

Directions:

Soak gelatin in some water (about 1 cup per 1 sheet of gelatin)

Heat the cream in a saucepan along with vanilla caviar and stevia sweetener; stir.

Add the egg yolks and continue to stir for further 2 - 3 minutes.

Remove from heat, add gelatin and stir well.

Pour vodka and stir again; allow the mixture to cool.

Pour the mixture in a container and refrigerate for at least 4 hours.

Remove the mixture in an ice cream maker; follow manufacturer's Instructions.

Or, pour the mixture in a freeze-safe container and freeze overnight.

Beat every 45 minutes with the mixture to prevent ice crystallization.

1Serve and enjoy!

Nutrition:

Calories: 118 Carbohydrates: 4g Proteins: 3g

Fat: 10g Fiber: 0g Sodium 67%

Traditional Spanish Cold Cream with Walnuts

Servings: 6

Preparation Time: 5 minutes

Cooking Time: 3 hours

Ingredients

3 cups of almond milk

3 cups of heavy cream

1 cup of ground walnuts

3/4 cup of natural sweetener (Stevia, Erythritol...etc.) or to taste

1 cinnamon stick

Directions:

Add all Ingredients from the list above in your Slow Cooker.

Cover and cook on HIGH for 3 hours.

During cooking stir several times with wooden spoon.

If your cream is too dense, add more almond milk.

Store cream in glass container and refrigerate for 4 hours.

Remove cream from the refrigerator 15 minutes before serving.

Nutrition:

Calories: 193 Carbohydrates: 5g

Proteins: 8g Fat: 20g

Fiber: 2g Sodium 30%

Chocolate Ice Cream

Servings: 6

Preparation Time: 15 minutes

Ingredients

1 can (15 oz) coconut milk

1/2 cup cocoa powder

1/4 cup natural sweetener (Stevia, Truvia, Erythritol...etc.)

1 tsp vanilla extract

Chopped nuts or shredded coconut For serving (optional)

Directions:

Combine all Ingredients in a bowl.

Use an electric mixer and beat the mixture until all Ingredients combine well.

Transfer the mixture in a freezer-safe bowl and freeze for 4 hours.

To prevent ice crystallization, beat the ice cream with the mixer every hour.

Serve garnished with sliced nuts or shredded coconuts.

Nutrition:

Calories: 204

Carbohydrates: 7g

Proteins: 4g

Fat: 21g

Fiber: 4.5g

Sodium 43%

Avocado and Strawberries Salad

Preparation time: 5 minutes

Cooking time: 0 minutes

Servings: 2

Ingredients:

1 banana, peeled and sliced

2 cups strawberries, halved

3 tablespoons mint, chopped

2 avocados, pitted and peeled

Directions:

In a bowl, combine the banana with the strawberries, mint and avocados, toss and serve cold.

Enjoy!

Nutrition:

calories 150, Fat 4,

Fiber 4,

Carbs 8,

Protein 6 Sodium 19%

Blueberry Cream

Preparation time: 5 minutes

Cooking time: 0 minutes

Servings: 1

Ingredients:

¾ cup blueberries

1 tablespoon low-

Fat peanut butter

¾ cup almond milk

1 banana, peeled

2 dates

Directions:

In a blender, combine the blueberries with peanut butter, milk, banana and dates, pulse well, divide into small cups and serve cold.

Enjoy!

Nutrition:

calories 120,

Fat 3,

Fiber 3,

Carbs 6, Protein 7 Sodium 9%

Apple Cupcakes

Preparation time: 10 minutes

Cooking time: 22 minutes

Servings: 12

Ingredients:

4 tablespoons coconut butter

½ cup natural applesauce

4 eggs

1 teaspoon vanilla extract

¾ cup almond flour

2 teaspoons cinnamon powder

½ teaspoon baking powder

1 apple, cored and sliced

Directions:

Heat up a pan with the butter over medium heat, add applesauce, vanilla and eggs, stir, heat up for 2 minutes, take off heat, cool down, add almond flour, baking powder and cinnamon, stir, divide into a lined cupcake pan, introduce in the oven at 350 degrees F and bake for 20 minutes.

Leave the cupcakes to cool down, divide between dessert plates and top with apple slices.

Enjoy!

Nutrition:

calories 200, Fat 4, Fiber 4,

Carbs 12, Protein 5 Sodium 52%

Cinnamon Apples

Preparation time: 10 minutes

Cooking time: 20 minutes

Servings: 4

Ingredients:

4 big apples, cored

4 tablespoons raisins

1 tablespoon cinnamon powder

Directions:

Stuff the apples with the raisins, sprinkle the cinnamon, arrange them in a baking dish, introduce in the oven at 375 degrees F, bake for 20 minutes and serve cold.

Enjoy!

Nutrition:

calories 200,

Fat 3,

Fiber 4,

Carbs 8,

Protein 5

Sodium 1%

Vanilla Pumpkin Bars

Preparation time: 10 minutes

Cooking time: 15 minutes

Servings: 14

Ingredients:

2 and ½ cups almond flour

½ teaspoon baking soda

1 tablespoon flax seed

3 tablespoons water

½ cup pumpkin flesh, mashed

¼ cup coconut sugar

2 tablespoons coconut butter

1 teaspoon vanilla extract

Directions:

In a bowl, mix flax seed with water and stir.

In another bowl, mix flour with, baking soda, flax meal, pumpkin, coconut sugar, coconut butter and vanilla, stir well, spread on a baking sheet, press well, bake in the oven at 350 degrees F for 15 minutes, leave aside to cool down, cut into bars and serve.

Enjoy!

Nutrition:

calories 210,

Fat 2,

Fiber 4,

Carbs 7,

Protein 8

Sodium 64%

Cold Cashew And Berry Cake

Preparation time: 5 hours

Cooking time: 0 minutes

Servings: 6

Ingredients:

For the crust:

½ cup dates, pitted

1 tablespoon water

½ teaspoon vanilla

½ cup almonds, chopped

For the cake:

2 and ½ cups cashews soaked overnight and drained

1 cup blackberries

¾ cup maple syrup

1 tablespoon coconut oil, melted

Directions:

In your food processor, mix dates with water, vanilla and almonds, pulse well, transfer this to a working surface, flatten it and press on the bottom of a round pan.

In your blender, mix maple syrup with coconut oil, cashews and blackberries, blend well, spread evenly over the crust, keep in the freezer for 5 hours, slice and serve.

Enjoy!

Nutrition: calories 230,

Fat 4, Fiber 4, Carbs 12,

Protein 8 Sodium 30%

Carrot And Mandarins Cold Cake

Preparation time: 3 hours

Cooking time: 0 minutes

Servings: 6

Ingredients:

3 carrots, grated

1/3 cup dates, pitted

4 mandarins, peeled

A handful walnuts, chopped

8 tablespoons coconut oil, melted

1 cup cashews, soaked for 2 hours

Juice of 2 lemons

2 tablespoons coconut sugar

2 tablespoons water

Directions:

In your food processor, mix carrots with dates, walnuts, mandarins and half of the coconut oil, blend very well, pour into a cake pan and spread well.

Add cashews to your food processor, also add lemon juice, stevia, water and the rest of the oil and blend some more.

Add this over the carrots mix, spread, keep in the fridge for 3 hours, slice and serve.

Enjoy!

Nutrition:

calories 170,

Fat 2,

Fiber 4,

Carbs 11,

Protein 8

Sodium 9%

Conclusion

If you want to improve your health to lose weight the DASH diet promotes a healthy diet which indicates you have to take the dash diet seriously, you will enjoy benefits like reduced high blood pressure, cholesterol and "type 2" diabetes

The DASH diet can be a perfect combination: a sensible diet to keep blood pressure levels under control and to lose pounds or maintain a healthy weight.

Dash diet lower risk of stroke and cardiovascular disease has been associated with the high consumption of vegetables and fruit typical of this diet.

The summary of Dash diet

It is a diet that keeps high blood pressure at bay

It can also be used to lose weight

It is similar to our Mediterranean diet

It should be customized according to needs

It limits saturated

Fats and salt in particular

Recommend to associate yourself with physical activity

The DASH diet without

Sodium loss or weight loss had a significant blood pressure lowering effect in virtually all subgroups.

This intervention adds to the current non-pharmacological approach to control hypertension.

Dietary Stop Hypertension (DASH) trials are rich in fruits, vegetables, low-fat dairy total and saturated fats, cholesterol, and sugar-containing products that effectively lower blood pressure in people with prehypertension.

The DASH diet leans heavily on vegetables, fruits, and whole grains. Fish and lean poultry are served moderately. Whole wheat flour is used instead of white flour. Using salt is discouraged. Instead, participants are encouraged to season foods with spices and herbs to add flavor without adding salt. DASH as a diet plan promotes the consumption of low-

Fat dairy, lean meat, fruits, and vegetables. It is literally a mix of old world and new world eating plans. It has been designed to follow old world diet principles to help eliminate new world health problems.

The carbohydrates are mainly made of plant fiber which the body does not easily digest and therefore cannot turn into stored fat. The plan is rich in good fats that make food taste good and help us feel fuller for a longer period of time.

Proteins are not forbidden but are geared more toward plant-based protein and not so much meat consumption.

When filling the plate for a meal, it is important that the food be attractive as well as tasty and nutritious. A wide variety of foods will make this plan much more interesting. Try to make choices that will offer a range of colors and textures. And remember that dessert is not off limits but should be based around healthy choices that include fresh fruit.

The DASH eating plans emphasis on vegetables, fruits, whole grains, and low-fat dairy products makes it an ideal plan for anyone looking to gain health through lowered blood pressure and a healthier heart. It is a heart healthy way of eating. The DASH plan has no specialized recipes or food plans. Daily caloric intake depends on a person's activity level and age. People who need to lose weight would naturally eat fewer calories.

The DASH diet's major focus is on grains, vegetables, and fruits because these foods are higher fiber foods and will make you feel full longer. Whole grains should be consumed six to eight times daily, vegetables four to six servings daily, and fruit four to five servings daily. Low-fat dairy is an important part of the diet and should be eaten two to three times daily. And there should be six or fewer servings daily of fish, poultry, and lean meat. The DASH diet does not limit red meat the way the Mediterranean diet does, but it still keeps it lean.

CPSIA information can be obtained
at www.ICGtesting.com
Printed in the USA
LVHW020827161120
671797LV00012B/569